ELEMENTAL ENERGY

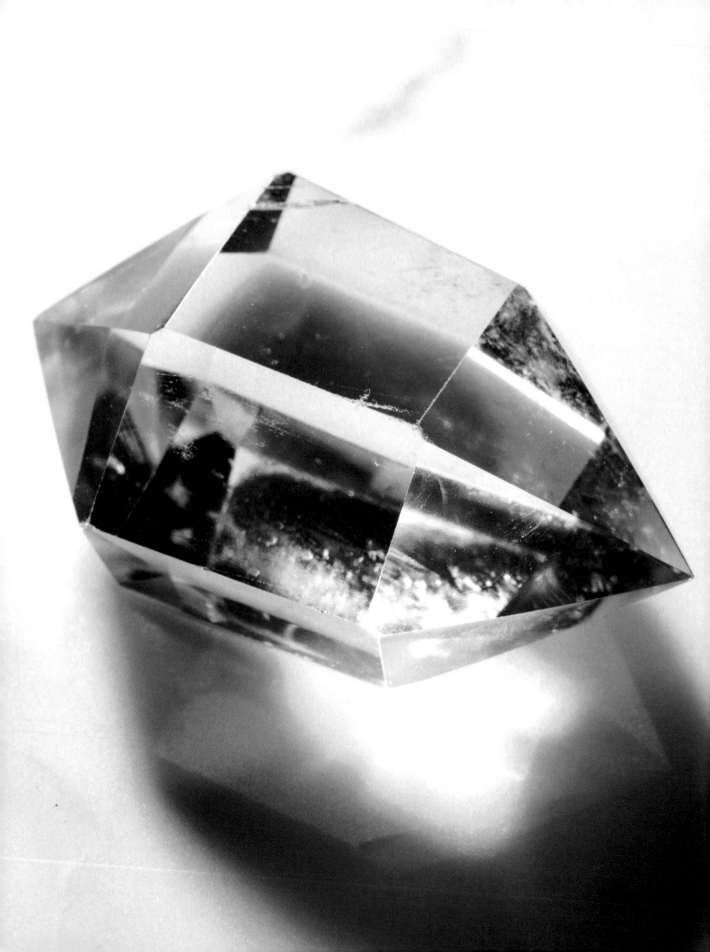

ELEMENTAL ENERGY

CRYSTAL AND GEMSTONE RITUALS
for a
BEAUTIFUL LIFE

KRISTIN PETROVICH

WITH MICHELE SHAPIRO

PHOTOGRAPHY BY ALICE GAO

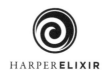

HARPER**ELIXIR**

This book is written as a source of information only. It is based on the research and observations of the author, who is not a medical doctor. The information in this book should by no means be considered a substitute for the advice of a qualified medical professional, who should always be consulted for any medical and health issues you may have. The author and the publisher expressly disclaim responsibility for any adverse effects arising from the use or application of information contained in this book.

HARPER**ELIXIR**

HarperCollins books may be purchased for educational, business, or sales promotional use. For information please e-mail the Special Markets Department at SPsales@harpercollins.com.

FIRST EDITION

Creative Direction and Book Design: Emily Wardwell
Photography: Alice Gao
Styling: Kira Corbin

Library of Congress Cataloging-in-Publication Data

Names: Petrovich, Kristin, author.
Title: Elemental energy : crystal and gemstone rituals for a beautiful life / Kristin Petrovich.
Description: First edition. | New York, NY : HarperElixir, 2016
Identifiers: LCCN 2016030269 (print) | LCCN 2016033226 (ebook) | ISBN 9780062428790 (hardback) | ISBN 9780062428837 (e-book)
Subjects: LCSH: Energy medicine. | Mind and body. | Healing. | BISAC: BODY, MIND & SPIRIT / Crystals. | BODY, MIND & SPIRIT / Healing. / General. | HEALTH & FITNESS / Alternative Therapies.
Classification: LCC RZ421 .P48 2016 (print) | LCC RZ421 (ebook) | DDC 615.8/51—dc23

LC record available at https://lccn.loc.gov/2016030269

ISBN 978-0-06-242879-0

16 17 18 19 20 QGT 10 9 8 7 6 5 4 3 2 1

In memory of my loving father,

Jon Alan Petrovich, whose passion, sense of humor,

and zest for life continues to inspire.

CONTENTS

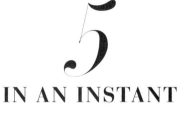

IN AN INSTANT

QUICK GEMSTONE AND CRYSTAL MASSAGES 85

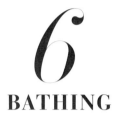

BATHING

GEMSTONE THERAPIES AND RITUALS 109

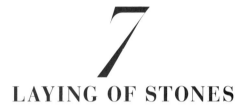

LAYING OF STONES

HEAD-TO-TOE ENERGY FLOW 135

REBALANCE, RESTORE, RECHARGE

GEMSTONE FACE AND BODY TREATMENTS 157

PERFECT RESONANCE

FINDING GEMSTONES FOR YOUR LIFESTYLE 187

INTRODUCTION

My fascination with gemstones started at an early age. It was not the presence of prismatic diamonds, sky-blue aquamarine, or even sunny citrine that grabbed my attention and held it for years to come. For me, it was the luster of pearls evoking a sense of allure and connection. Long before my daughter, Kristin, and I ever pondered the concept of a luxury skincare line infused with the energy of pearls, gemstones, and precious minerals, I gravitated toward these iridescent spheres. From that first introduction, I just loved how smooth they felt between my fingers and against my skin.

As a child growing up in Indiana near Lake Michigan, my mother had a particular strand of pearls that magically turned any outfit she wore—from a black cocktail dress to a white button-down blouse and capris—into pure elegance. The necklace had been a gift from my grandmother, and I envisioned it one day being passed down to me.

It wasn't until my teenage years that pearls began to serve a newfound purpose. My mother, who looked far younger than her age, shared her secret: she would sometimes sleep with a strand of pearls around her neck, and, as she explained, the body's natural oils would capture the inner luster of the pearls. She encouraged me to follow the same ritual, and most mornings my skin looked brighter, as did my mental outlook.

Before Kristin and I launched our holistic skincare line, själ, in 2001, a cosmetic chemist with whom Kristin and I were working suggested that we include pearl extract in our products to help promote luminosity, brightening, and overall clarity. I was curious as to why our chemist felt pearls had these effects on the skin. Her response confirmed my original insights—that pearls are actually gemstones, and gemstones naturally radiate energy.

From yearning for my mother's pearl necklace to the birth of Kristin's and my skincare line, it was now clear why I gravitated toward pearls and gemstones.

When I began my journey with gemstones and crystals, I had just moved to California. Kristin had left for college, and my husband was traveling the globe. Anything but a New Age hippie, I was still conservative in my views; however, I felt there was something missing in life. After catching a feng shui expert on *The Oprah Winfrey Show*, I decided to contact the expert so she would work her magic in our home and my husband's office—unbeknownst to him, of course. She suggested I buy a few affordable gemstones to keep

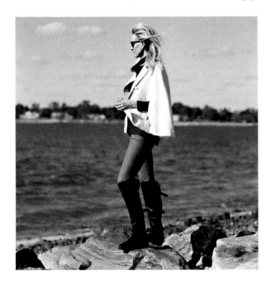

around the house and hide a handful in my husband's office drawers to emit positive energy while deflecting the negative. I went onto a New Age website and ordered a kit containing one each of red, orange, yellow, green, blue, and purple stones. I decided to put a set on my nightstand because I wanted them nearby, though I didn't know why.

I felt an immediate connection with the purple amethyst, much in the same way I had experienced with pearls. I later learned that purple stones resonate with the Crown chakra at the top of the head—the center for trust, devotion, inspiration, and positivity, which is also the center for deeper connection with ourselves and the divine. It's no wonder that by simply closing my eyes and holding the stone for a few minutes every day while visualizing its deep purple color, I felt calmer and more connected to a higher power.

Although Kristin is usually the one in the know when it comes to the latest fashion, food, and health trends, I was actually the first to view gemstones as tools that connect the mind, body, and spirit in a way I'd never experienced.

When Kristin learned of my newfound interest in gemstones and crystals, she was skeptical to say the least. She returned home from college and spotted the collection on my nightstand. "What are these tchotchkes doing in here? They're hideous," I recall her saying. My family was convinced I had lost my mind. And I wasn't 100 percent sure that that wasn't the case.

Right around the same time, during a routine visit, my doctor discovered that I had several cysts that were cause for concern and that would require surgery. Needless to say, this weighed heavily on me. After my diagnosis, my husband, Jon, and I took a trip to

Sedona, Arizona. As I hiked amid the stunningly impressive and humbling red rocks of Sedona, which, like gemstones, were formed over millions of years, I felt more connected to the earth than I ever had. I asked the universe for a sign—a physical sign—that my journey with gemstones and their ability to heal and protect was valid. I needed to know that the tingling I felt coming from the stones and moving through my body wasn't all in my head.

I never had to have those cysts removed. At my next doctor's visit, there was no trace of them—none! Miraculously, they had all dissolved. My doctor couldn't believe it. Nor could I. The changes in me weren't just physical. My doctor noticed that there was something different about my aura. "What have you been doing?" she asked. What she must have picked up on was how much more comfortable I had become with my decisions and in my new life path.

Now if I could only get Kristin to be open to the possibilities. After graduating from college, she headed straight to New York City to pursue a career in fashion. Almost immediately, she started working as an assistant for several top stylists, and her days were long. As a mom, I worried about her burning the candle at both ends. But she insisted on doing

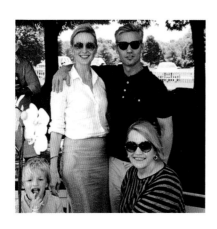

everything in her power to forge a career, knowing that if she turned down a job, somebody else would swoop right in to take it. The stress took its toll, and eventually she felt so run-down, she could barely get out of bed. I sent her a small purple amethyst cluster, which I am sure she dismissed.

It wasn't until she returned home from a photo shoot one evening with a fever so high she could barely move that she plopped into bed, fumbled for the stone, and placed it near her head while she drifted off. The next morning, she felt almost 100 percent better. But something strange had happened to the stone: each stem of the purple crystal cluster was black at the top, as if it had absorbed her pain as well as the heat from her body.

That was the turning point. She had realized that the gemstone's power to heal wasn't just New Age hokum. In fact, it wasn't new at all, since for thousands of years, various cultures, from the ancient Egyptians, Greeks, and Romans in the West to the Hindi and Chinese cultures in the East, had witnessed stones' protective and healing powers. Shamans and medicine men used them as tools to connect to the divine, and century after century, great thinkers and physicians have continued to understand stones' abilities to connect us with the earth and the heavens.

Kristin spent the next few years trying to understand what had transpired that night. Like I had done for years, she now studied and experimented with Eastern practices including Chinese, Tibetan, ayurvedic, homeopathic, and vibrational medicines. She visited

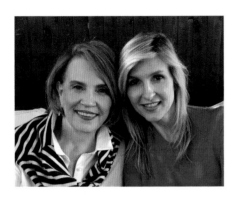

herbalists, holistic medical practitioners, integrative nutritionists, and crystal healers to better comprehend the philosophy behind why energy is considered by many to be the best medicine (with no refills required or side effects).

When she began the research in her late twenties, Kristin was drawn to rose quartz, perhaps because it's known as the love stone. Now she swears by black hematite (the same stone responsible for the deeply colored top layer of red rock in Sedona) to keep her grounded as she juggles running a business with raising my rambunctious five-year-old grandson, Van, and finding time for date nights with her husband, James.

I'm over-the-moon happy that Kristin has written a book for those like her, who lead lives with a constant undercurrent of stress and anxiety as well as other environmental influences that take a toll on their health and well-being.

With her impeccable taste and solid understanding of the mineral world, Kristin is the perfect ambassador to reinterpret age-old traditions using gemstones and minerals for today's time-pressed lifestyle. Her gift to you: dozens of DIY treatments and simple techniques—mini massages, soothing and energizing baths, face and body treatments, and the ancient stones-laying rituals. Some take just a few minutes. Others permit you to carve out thirty or forty minutes of "me" time one or more days a week.

In addition, she'll let you know the essential stones and tools you need to get started on your gemstone journey. Just as my mother eventually passed her strand of pearls down to me, I've been fortunate enough to pass along my love and knowledge of gemstones to my daughter. I know she is excited to share the discoveries we have made together over the past two decades (and continue to make every day). We hope that you, too, will find the elements of energy and pass them on to those you love.

We are truly one.

—KAREN PETROVICH,
COFOUNDER, själ skincare

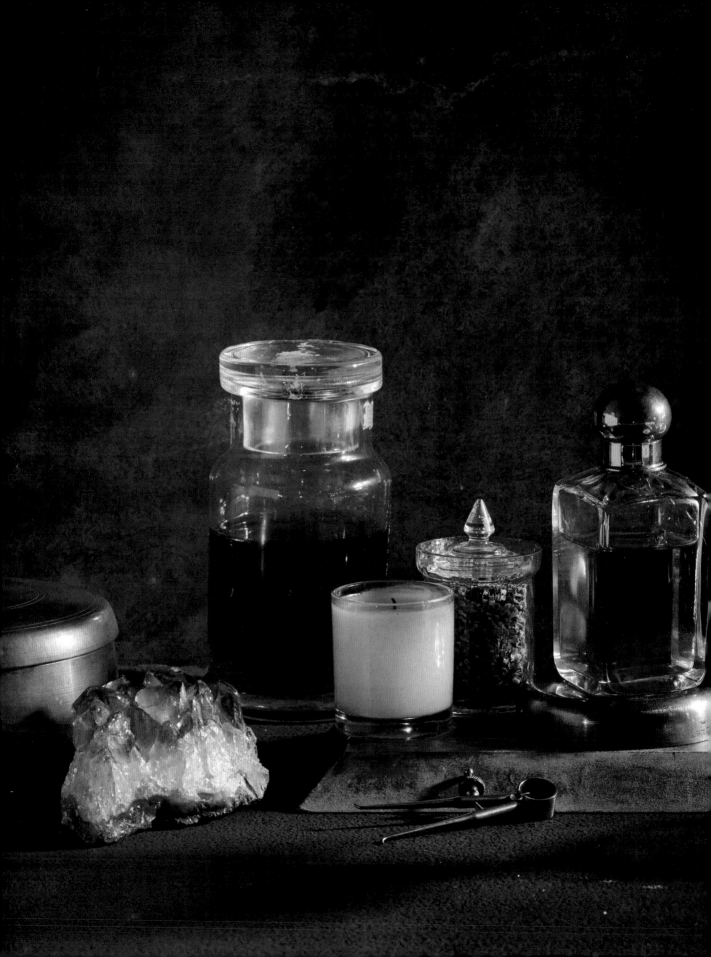

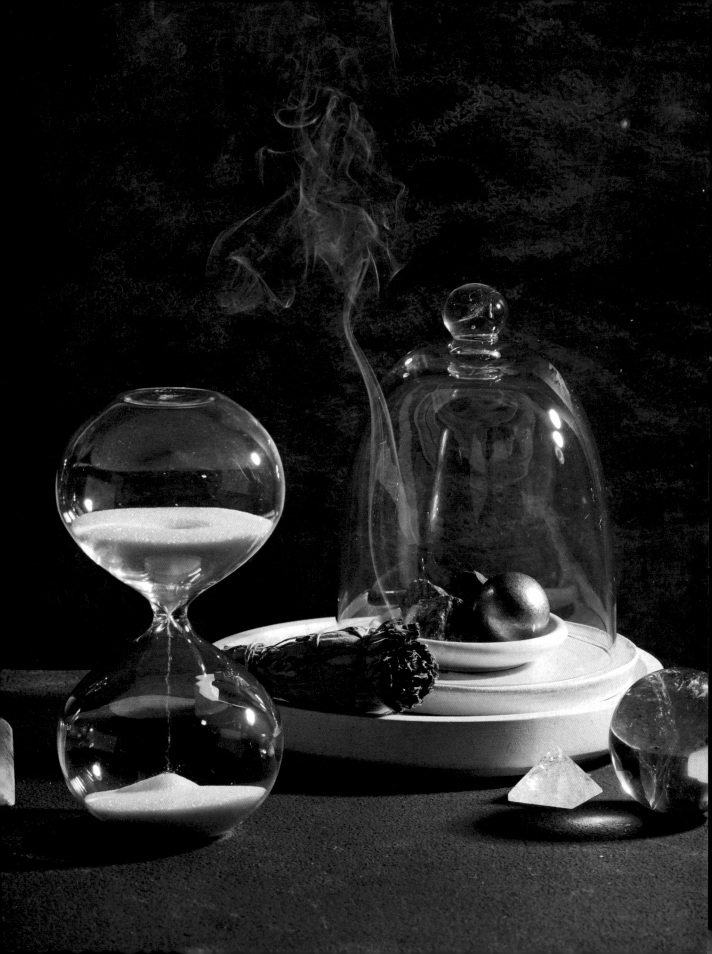

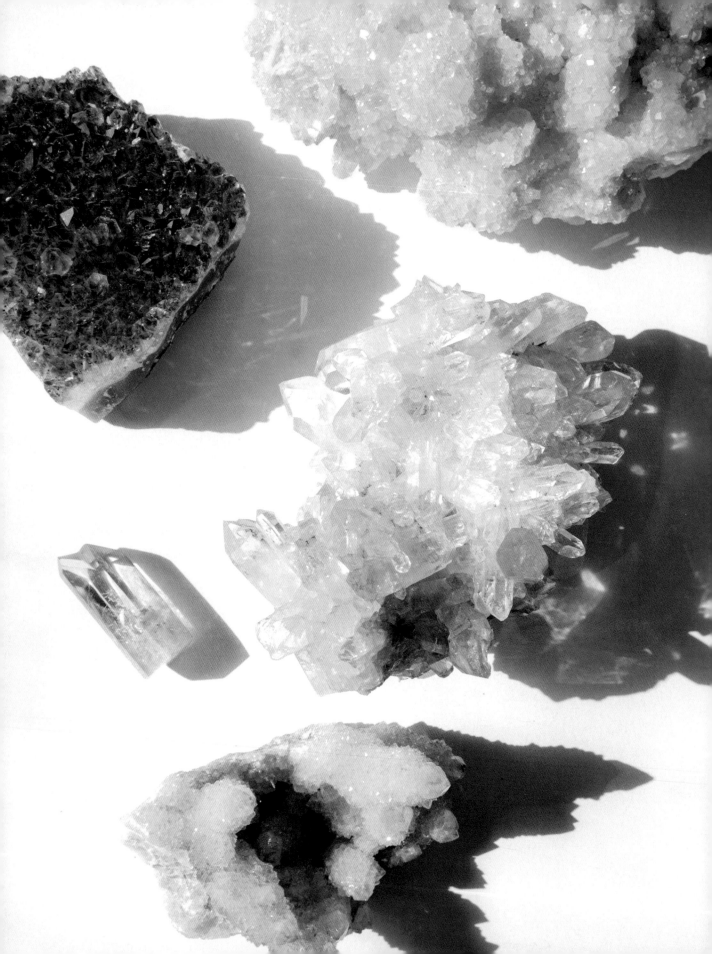

1

GOOD VIBRATIONS

CRYSTAL AND GEMSTONE ENERGY

Trust me, I know that at first it's hard to imagine that crystals and gemstones, as beautiful as they are, possess a vibrant healing energy. I know, because I used to find the idea completely far-fetched myself. Still, when you think about the fact that stones originate deep within the earth's crust and that we have a natural harmony with the earth, it begins to make sense. But don't take my word for it. Belief in the healing power of these stones dates back thousands of years to the earliest civilizations. Ancient cultures embraced the idea that the wide variety of stones they mined had talismanic powers. In other words, when crystals and gems were worn, carried, or pulverized and rubbed on people's skin, they were thought to protect against everything from disease to evil spirits.

Not surprisingly, holistically inclined Eastern cultures were among the first to explore the medicinal and therapeutic properties of crystals and gems. Transcriptions from the earliest Indian Vedic texts and Chinese medical books mention crystals and gemstones. Ayurveda, the Vedic tradition of naturopathic medicine, describes in great detail how to prepare elixirs, pastes, and powders made from gems to balance out the body's energies, or *doshas,* while the Chinese used crystals and gemstones in various types of pastes, powders, and solutions for topical application. Above all other stones, they attributed curative powers to jade, which they used to treat asthma and illnesses related to blood.

WHICH CAME FIRST?

The terms *mineral, crystal,* and *gemstone* are often used interchangeably, yet there are distinct differences. Here's how to tell them apart:

MINERALS

Minerals are the basic building blocks of the earth. Currently there are over four thousand identified minerals, and dozens more are discovered each year. Society depends on minerals as sources of metals, like iron (Fe), copper (Cu), gold (Au), silver (Ag), zinc (Zn), nickel (Ni), and aluminum (Al). The general definition of a mineral, which is composed of atoms, encompasses the following criteria: it forms in nature on its own, it's a solid rather than a liquid or a gas, and it has a definite chemical composition expressed by a chemical formula, as well as a characteristic crystalline structure (atoms are arranged within the mineral in a specific ordered manner). If a substance satisfies some but not all of the parts of the definition (opal, for example, lacks the crystalline structure), it's called a mineraloid.

CRYSTALS

Most minerals occur naturally as crystals, which have an orderly internal pattern of atoms. The shape of a crystal mirrors that internal arrangement. As crystals grow, differences in temperature and chemical composition cause variations. When many crystals grow near one another, they mesh together to form a mass. Granite, for instance, is made up of tiny crystals. The internal arrangement of atoms also determines a crystal's color. Many minerals, like quartz, are colorless in their pure state, but crystals occur in a range of colors from pink to brown to deep purple, depending on the number and type of impurities in their structure.

GEMSTONES

Gemstones are crystals that have been cut and polished. Jewelers select certain crystals to cut into gems because of their extraordinary color, flashes of color (known as "fire"), and hardness. In general, any attractive, relatively flawless crystal is fodder to be cut into a gem. However, the majority of gems used in jewelry today come from about fifteen different crystals. Size, beauty, rarity, and durability are the basic criteria that determine a gem's value, though a rich and interesting history can add to that worth.

By the Middle Ages, every advanced
civilization knew of stones' healing properties, and
many books were published on the subject.

The medical and mythical appeal of crystals and gems thrived in Western cultures as well. Ancient Egyptian men and women wore amulets, protective charms carved from colorful stones such as purple amethyst, red jasper, and orange carnelian. They believed so strongly in the stones' protective powers that they insisted on being buried with them to ensure their departed soul's safe travel to the next life.

Today this thinking sounds strange and more than a little superstitious. However, long before the first celebrity ever walked a red carpet decked out, the association of gemstones with wealth and power enhanced their amuletic potency. Pharaohs wore headdresses lined with dark malachite to help them rule wisely. Others wore bloodred stones, such as rubies, to keep from getting wounded, or crushed sky-blue lapis lazuli, a symbol of creation and rebirth, into powder and rubbed it into the crowns of their heads to extract spiritual impurities.

In ancient Greece, crystals and gemstones were held in equally high esteem. In fact, the word "crystal" is thought to be derived from the Greek word *krustallos*, or "ice," and many ancients believed clear quartz crystals were eternal ice sent from the heavens. The great philosopher Aristotle spoke of the power of healing stones, and the Romans followed suit, carrying crystal and gemstone fragments to ward off sickness and ill fortune.

Dating back to around 450 BCE, the biblical stories of the Old Testament underscored the significance of crystals and gemstones as symbols of strength and divinity. And, once again, they were shown to protect—Zircon was the name of the guardian angel sent to watch over Adam and Eve in the Garden of Eden, and in the book of Exodus, there is a description of a breastplate Moses gave to his brother, the high priest Aaron, that contains twelve sacred gemstones.

By the Middle Ages, every advanced civilization knew of stones' healing properties, and many books were published on the subject. *Natural History,* in which Roman historian Pliny the Elder (ca. 23–79 CE) discusses the properties of various stones and gems categorized by color, durability, and origin, became the basis for knowledge about rocks and minerals throughout the period. Marbod, the Bishop of Rennes (ca. 1035–1123 CE) as well as a poet, later wrote the *Book of Stones,* or *Liber lapidum,* which describes—in verse—the various medicinal qualities of sixty gems and minerals including diamond, topaz, sapphire or lapis lazuli, and coral. (Coral, like amber and pearl, is among a small group of organic gemstones created by living things.)

Shortly thereafter in the twelfth century, a woman far ahead of her time, the German Benedictine abbess and mystic Hildegard von Bingen, wrote the comprehensive work *Physika*. In the book, she boldly suggested that medicine needed a holistic orientation, and that physical and spiritual disorders couldn't be isolated from environmental influences. Among the treatments she suggested were ancient rituals such as placing stones on parts of the anatomy and prescribing concoctions made from minerals and the essences of gemstones for specific illnesses.

Crystal and gemstone healing gained even more momentum during the Renaissance when, in his treatise on minerals, physician and philosopher Philippus Aureolus Theophrastus Bombastus von Hohenheim (aka Paracelsus) made a distinction between chemical formulas and the elemental powers residing within stones.

Eventually, the gradual development of modern medicine after the Renaissance led to an erosion of previously held beliefs. Crystals and gemstones continued to grace the necks of the British aristocracy and the rings of cardinals, but their healing properties were all but forgotten by many Western cultures over time.

Fortunately, integrative medicine—and subsequently a renewed interest in the therapeutic use of gemstones and crystals—has experienced a renaissance of sorts in recent years as more and more people realize the potential of alternative or complementary practices that have their roots in Eastern medicine. Stones can be magical, mystical, *and* medicinal. They have an energy, an electricity of sorts, which is believed to be transformative and healing.

MY JOURNEY WITH CRYSTALS AND GEMSTONES

Harnessing the power of gemstones and crystals was not our original intention when my mother and I decided to start our skincare line, själ. Our goal was to create products that integrated ancient Eastern healing practices with the latest Western innovations. We believed the answer lay in the synergy of these two very different practices. But what could be the link or connection? As we began researching Western biotechnology and degenera-

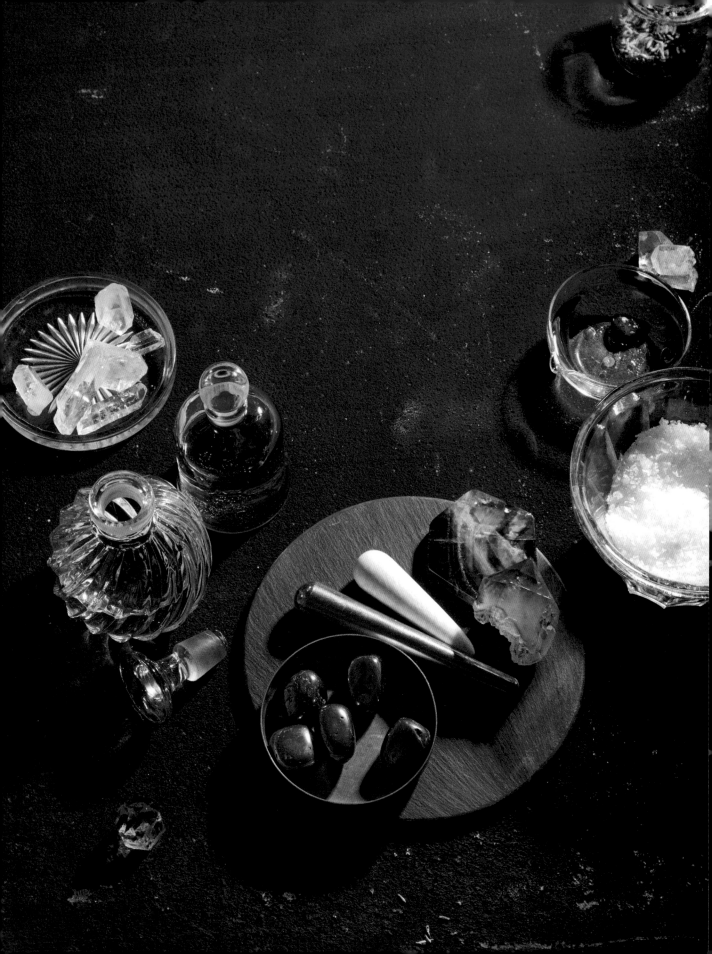

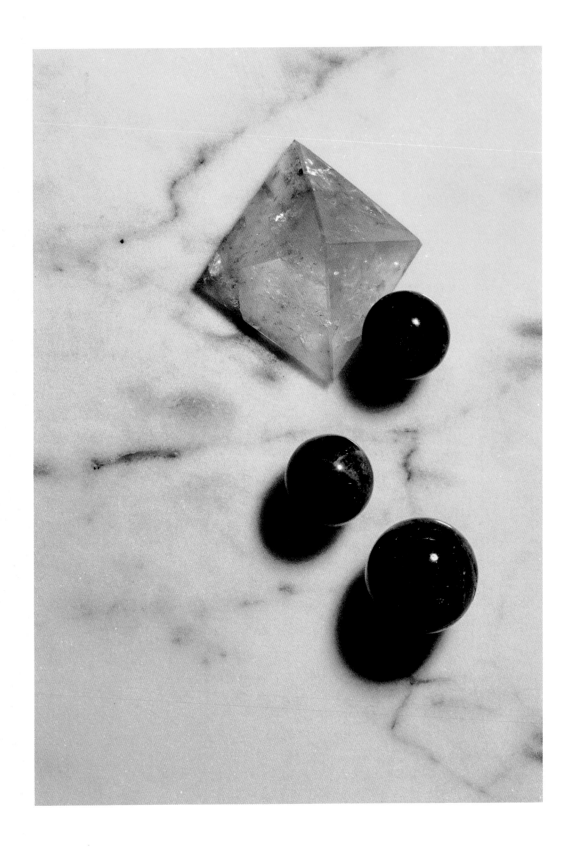

My mom had started collecting a colorful
array of small and large crystals and gemstones
back when I was in college. She loved searching
for them when she traveled with my dad . . .

tive aging diseases, we came across research on the experimental use of nanoparticles of precious metals such as gold and platinum to target cancer cells with laserlike precision.

Could precious metals also help to repair damaged skin cells? A chemist we were working with on our formulations confirmed that gold and platinum, as well as silver and copper, have the ability to boost cellular productivity, improving skin's elasticity and firmness while also acting as natural antibacterials and antimicrobials. What's more, they are known for their regenerative properties. We had found our connection—precious metals that have been used for centuries in ancient medicines were now being used in modern-day science.

At first, my mom and I imagined having to melt down all of our fine jewelry to create the first batch of products. Fortunately, we discovered a way to incorporate precious metals into our creams, serums, and masks through the use of colloidals, which are suspended microscopic particles of gold, silver, and platinum in a liquid mixture. We were ecstatic to be able to use colloidals in our products, as they not only complemented our ingredients but enhanced the products' performance.

Almost a year later, a holistic practitioner suggested we take the products to the next level by incorporating energy into our products through the use of gemstones. We considered ourselves to be open but even this idea seemed a bit out there. . . . After all, we wanted our products to be taken seriously, and this wasn't something we wanted to highlight in the world of clinical science. After some consideration, we figured we had nothing to lose, and, at the very least, if all matter has energy, why not program the products with something as positive and cool as gemstone energy? Besides, we were already using gold and silver, so why not incorporate gemstones for their natural energistic properties?

My mom had started collecting a colorful array of small and large crystals and gemstones back when I was in college. She loved searching for them when she traveled with my dad and often returned home with unusual stones that were at once souvenirs and soul soothers. Initially I was skeptical of her stones' ability to do anything other than look pretty, but over time I opened my mind as well as my heart to their mysterious powers and amassed a small collection of my own. While my mom swore that meditating with an

THE RAINBOW CONNECTION

Below are some examples of gemstones and crystals and the impurities that provide their brilliant colors.

GEMSTONE	COLOR	HOST CRYSTAL	IMPURITY
ruby	red	corundum	chromium
emerald	green	beryl	chromium
garnet	red	calcium aluminosilicate	iron
topaz	yellow	aluminum fluorosilicate	iron
tourmaline	pink-red	calcium lithium boroaluminosilicate	manganese
turquoise	blue-green	copper phosphoaluminate	copper

amethyst made her more open and intuitive, for me it was all about rose quartz (aka the love stone). When I got bold enough to purchase my first stone, I felt drawn to the glass case containing dozens of rose quartz specimens. I asked the salesperson if I could hold one in my hand—I felt an immediate connection with it, which materialized as a gentle tingling sensation up my arm. I bought the stone on the spot and never looked back. I knew little about stones at the time, but I slept with this stone, I bathed with it, and I displayed it on my coffee table. I couldn't believe how much I naturally gravitated toward this stone. I was in my late twenties at the time and open to finding love. (I can't guarantee that the pink stone brought my husband, James, and me together, but we did get married two years later.)

Though my mother and I lived on opposite coasts during those years—she in Los Angeles, I in New York City—we'd both started experimenting with numerous Eastern healing practices, from acupuncture to Reiki to reflexology. I'd experienced firsthand how powerful these treatments could be for grounding and centering me on days when my mind was ten steps ahead of my body, or revitalizing me when I felt drained both emotionally and creatively. The latter was exactly the case when I hit a wall after a year of working 24/7 as a styling assistant. When I explained to a doctor of integrative medicine how run-down and exhausted I felt, he said he'd seen several women my age complaining of similar symptoms. After a thorough exam, he prescribed some supplements and strongly urged me to try acupuncture and jotted down the address of a practitioner in Chinatown. Being poked and prodded with needles sounded anything but relaxing—in fact, it sounded downright scary. I made and canceled three appointments before mustering up the courage to go. When I arrived and saw that the only thing separating me from the patient on the table beside mine was a thin muslin curtain, I almost ran right out the door.

I'm so glad I didn't. I barely felt the dozen or so needles the Chinese doctor inserted in my neck, back, and hands. But I was amazed at how, after around twenty minutes of lying motionless on the table, I began to feel miniature lightning bolts gently moving through my body breaking up any blockages and tension. I was so relaxed, I actually fell asleep, and then I woke up feeling as if I'd slept for a week.

Similarly, my mom had experienced a deep sense of tranquility by meditating with gemstones and crystals at home. It's interesting that our different needs (mine more physical, hers more spiritual) led us to the same conclusion: integrating the best of the East and West is key for living a healthy and productive lifestyle. This became the driving force behind our brand as well as the ethos by which we continue to live.

ELEMENTAL ENERGY

Before we founded själ, my mother and I intuitively accepted the restorative powers of crystals and gemstones—after all, we experienced their healing effects in our daily lives. But once we started formulating our products, I knew I would have to understand more about *how* crystals and gemstones work. In other words, what's behind crystal and gemstone energy? As I have learned, that answer can be condensed into two words: *origins* and *oscillations*. Once I began to delve into the incredibly prolonged process of how crystals and gemstones form, as well as each crystal's unique (and uniquely complex) internal structure that leads it to vibrate continuously at a consistently high frequency, it became clear to me why gemstones and crystals have long held intrinsic appeal for people from all walks of life—from kings to clerics and medics to mystics—and why they possess intense concentrations of energy.

ENERGY SOURCE 1
THE MOVEMENT OF MAGMA

The next time you're feeling old, think about this: most gemstones and crystals form due to forces that have been at work for billions of years. Yes, *billions*. That's how long it takes for bubbling hot magma from the earth's core to push its way up to the crust, forming minerals, which in turn form interlocking crystals. The finest and rarest of those crystals are then cut and polished into gemstones. (See "Which Came First?," page 4.)

WHAT MAKES QUARTZ AND OTHER MINERALS A GO-TO FOR TECHNOLOGIES WE RELY ON 24/7?

Crystals that acquire an electric charge when compressed, twisted, or distorted are said to be piezoelectric. Through the piezoelectric effect, mechanical energy can be converted or transduced into electromagnetic energy, and vice versa. With this in mind, it's not difficult to imagine that crystals may be capable of transforming or amplifying other forms of energy that may not yet have been detected by scientific instruments.

A number of critical factors—the time it takes for the magma to travel from core to crust, its temperature, the amount of pressure it endures, and how long it takes to cool down once its journey is complete—influence what type of crystal or gemstone results from the presence of a single mineral or a combination of them. Some crystals and gemstones grow inside gas bubbles after magma reaches the surface. Others form when water and other liquids evaporate. Additionally, as the earth's crust shifts, new elements can be introduced that affect a crystal's chemical makeup, color, and growth pattern. It's no wonder there are over 130 species of minerals that have been cut into gems!

Since the magma is constantly in motion throughout the formation process, the rocks in which the minerals form are storehouses of energy. Remember that tingling up my arm I felt when I first held a rose quartz in my hand? At the time I thought, *It must be all in my head*. But the more I read about the basic principles of energy from a physicist's perspective, the surer I was that what I had experienced in the store that day was actually a transfer of electrical energy from the stone to me. You see, physicists define energy as moving something against a force, such as gravity. In physics, energy can be transformed into another sort of energy, the two most common of which are kinetic (something moves) and potential (something's poised to move). However, it cannot be created or destroyed. In other words, energy has always existed in one form or another. If you take into account the kinetically driven origins of crystals and gems, it's easy to view rose quartz or any other

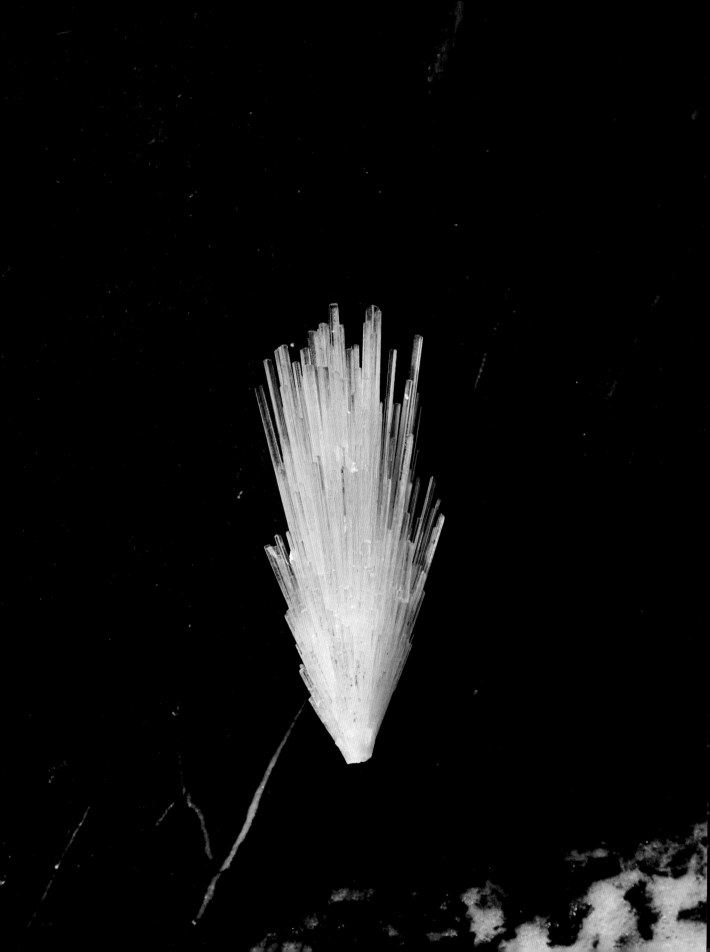

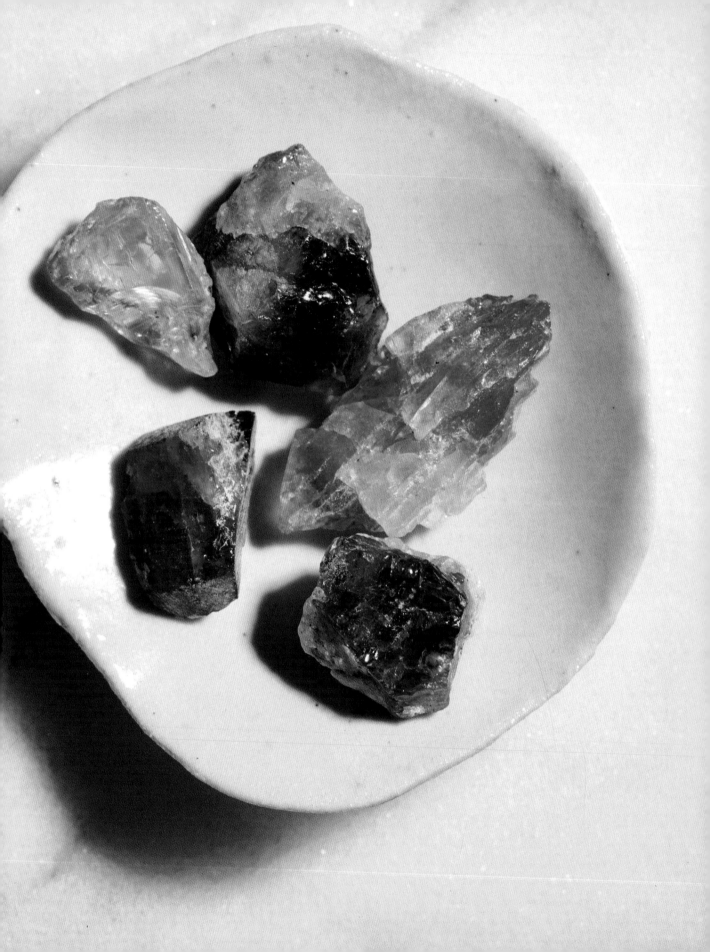

stone as a source of potential energy that transforms into electrical energy when it comes in contact with a heat source—in this case, my skin.

While not all crystals and gemstones originate from rock composed of magma, their creation always involves some sort of seismic shift or perpetual movement. Crystals can form when water rushes over rocks and carries bits and pieces away into lakes, oceans, or streams until the fragments form layers that eventually harden into sedimentary rock, or when the earth's crust buckles and folds, ultimately changing existing crystal structures in rocks. The crystals and gems that form in these metamorphic conditions tend to be pretty small.

ROCK STARS

The rocks in which the plethora of gemstones and crystals form fall into one of three main categories: igneous rocks, sedimentary rocks, and metamorphic rocks. Here's how each rock type fosters the formation of brilliant crystals and gemstones:

IGNEOUS

Home to: Diamond, topaz, kunzite, and spinel

How gems form: Liquid magma composed of molten rock and lava wells up within the earth until intense pressure builds, forcing the liquid rock to the surface. Over time, the interlocking gemstones and crystals grow within these rocks. The minerals present, the cooling time, and the environment all affect the way in which these gemstones and crystals form.

SEDIMENTARY

Home to: Sapphires, rubies, and quartz

How gems form: Rock fragments near the earth's surface are washed into riverbeds and seabeds. Over time, layers of the fragments, along with mud and other organic and inorganic elements, are compacted into hard rock.

METAMORPHIC

Home to: Jadeite, peridot, and some types of emeralds

How gems form: Recrystallization is caused by intense pressure and high temperatures, transforming the composition of a rock deep within the earth's crust, or through direct contact with hot magma.

So how do crystals become the large, well-formed geodes you see on display in museums? It's all a matter of how much space they have to branch out; the larger the rock cavity in which they form, the larger the crystal.

ENERGY SOURCE 2
COMPOSITION AND STRUCTURE

Given the origins of most crystals and gemstones from deep within the earth, I'm not at all surprised that certain stones have the ability to make me feel grounded. But why are others able to lift my spirits and deepen my thinking, or even help me develop a direct connection to a higher power?

The answer quite possibly lies in their internal vibrations. These vibrations—or oscillations—result from the back-and-forth motion of particles within the stone, which are triggered by the tremendous force and pressure involved in their formation. Although the magma eventually morphs from liquid chemical "soup" into solids that house crystals and gems, the stones' tumultuous history leads them to vibrate consistently at frequencies that tend to be higher than other matter, including our own. They are constantly oscillating, whereas our energy levels fluctuate.

Crystals and gemstones are super-charged for two indisputable reasons: their unique chemical makeup and their crystalline structure, or "lattice." The two go hand in hand since, without one or the other, the minerals that make up crystals and gemstones would end up as far less glamorous rocks. Instead, the lattice structure of quartz, beryl, and diamonds, among other stones, provides great stability and regularity of flow of any energies that move through it. While crystals tend to be the workhorses and gemstones the "show horses," crystals are no less powerful in terms of frequency, which refers to how often the particles of the medium vibrate. In fact, because quartz crystals vibrate like clockwork, they are often incorporated into watches to provide highly accurate measurements of time, and man-made crystals with structures identical to natural ones are used to power laptops, cell phones, and other electronics.

The chemical makeup (or composition) of crystals and gemstones can be expressed by a chemical formula. Diamond consists of carbon, for instance, while emerald is a beryllium aluminum silicate and peridot is a magnesium iron silicate. Interestingly, diamond, the most precious of all gemstones, and graphite (pencil lead) have the same chemical composition: pure carbon. The only difference is that diamonds are formed under greater pressure and at higher temperatures.

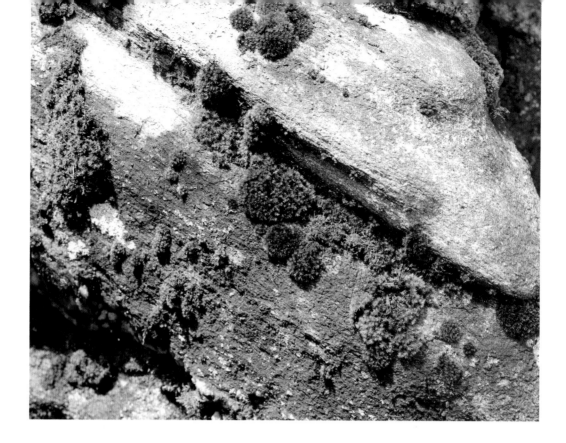

From a wellness standpoint, different compositions allow for different energies, properties, and characteristics. For example, hematite is red iron oxide (Fe_2O_3), which is thought to aid circulation and ground and support organs. (Perhaps the iron that the stone contains is what made ancient Greek soldiers feel so invincible when they crushed and rubbed the stones on their skin before heading into battle.)

The other driving force behind crystal energy is its unique structure. Be they minerals, salt, or snowflakes, all crystals have an orderly internal arrangement of atoms that's somewhat akin to that neat-freak roommate you had in college who folded one shirt on top of the other into a perfect pile. These repeated patterns occur within the basic atomic structure and reflect the pattern of faces of the crystal. With larger stones, you can see the characteristic symmetry simply by looking at it. This variety and perfection of form and symmetry has led geologists, gemologists, technologists, and theologians to respect and revere crystals as a true natural wonder.

I share their sense of constant discovery and fascination with the power of crystals and gemstones, whether I am wearing them or viewing them as conduits to physical, mental, and spiritual wellness. I'm excited to act as your guide in the chapters that follow and to lead you on a personal journey to discover which stones you gravitate toward—and help explain why—as well as providing hundreds of ideas for incorporating crystals and gemstones into your life in ways that are both meaningful and memorable.

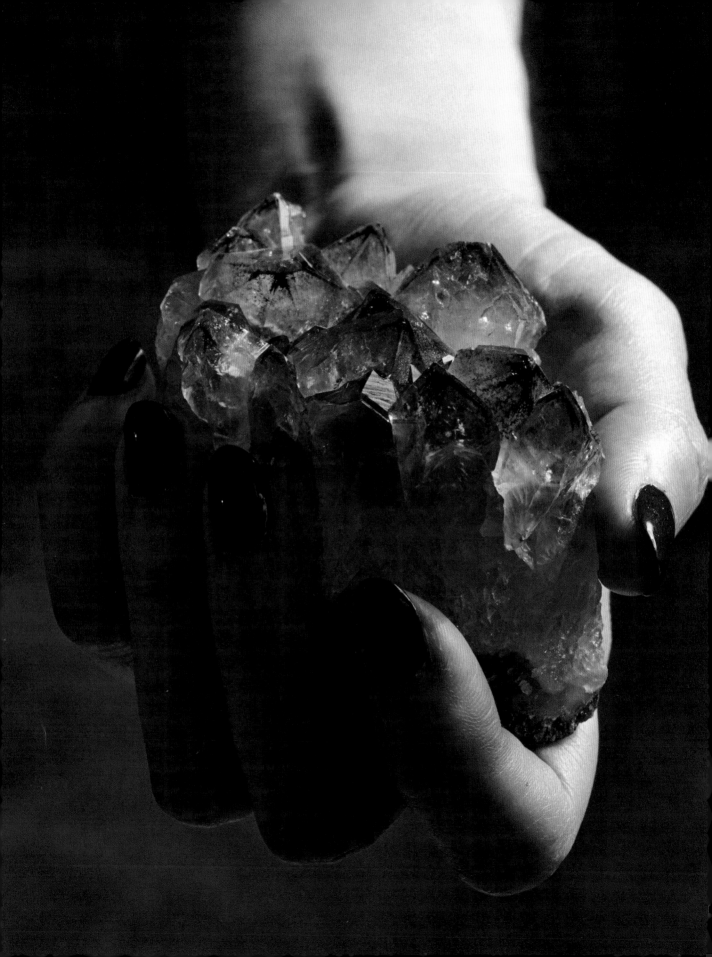

2

NATURAL HARMONY

WHY WE RESPOND TO GEMSTONES

A s humans, we intuitively accept that we have energy. When our energy's high, life is good. We aim to eat healthy, get up early to excercise, generate creative ideas for business and personal projects, cross to-dos off our lists, and turn chaos into order. On the flip side, when our energy flags or wavers, we can feel of little use until we renew, recharge, or reboot. But what exactly are we getting at when we use a metaphor like "recharge"? After all, we're not electronic gadgets that come with charging cables and power cords . . . or are we?

THE BODY AS AN ENERGY SYSTEM

Chances are you've never heard of Robert O. Becker. I hadn't either until I began my deep dive into researching crystal and gemstone healing properties for my business. Born in 1923, Becker became an orthopedic surgeon and professor who researched electrophysiology, the study of the electrical properties of biological cells and tissues. He conducted groundbreaking research that suggests living organisms and animals possess a direct current of electric charge (aka a DC electric field), which has the potential to help them heal everything from bone fractures to heart conditions, just as it had helped hydras grow new heads in his lab and salamander amputees regenerate lost limbs.

While working for the Veterans Administration, Dr. Becker explored the regenerative powers of these internal currents. He documented that open wounds emit an electric charge, much like wires that have been cut, and he experimented with the veterans themselves to observe the differences in the way they healed by means of their internal power sources. In 1985, Dr. Becker compiled his extensive findings in a book called *The Body Electric*. Despite his breakthroughs, he received few accolades. In fact, his funding was often pulled before he even completed his studies, because his theories were viewed in a less than favorable light by the medical and pharmaceutical industries.

But from my perspective, Dr. Becker was a true pioneer. His work has helped me to better understand why my body responds to the electrical properties in crystals and gemstones. It's almost as if when I place a stone on a particular body part or keep it near me in a room, its strong electrical charge jump-starts my energy in the same way a jumper cable would work on a car battery—it gets the electrical current moving through the body's "stalled" circuitry.

By thinking of the human body as an electric entity, it's easier to understand why we respond—not only emotionally but also physically—to the electrical properties inherent in crystals and gemstones, as well as how we can use that knowledge to manipulate our internal currents to maximize energy flow.

There's another possible reason we resonate with crystal and gemstone energy: research over the years suggests our bodies are filled with oscillating solid and liquid crystals. The highly ordered and neatly organized structures resemble those of mineral crystals and many gemstones found in the earth. But how extensive have scientists determined these structures to be, and what is their role in getting, and keeping, us feeling energetic and alive?

In trying to answer those questions, I came across the work of Dr. Mae-Wan Ho, a Hong Kong–born geneticist and biochemist who now resides in London. She approaches Western medicine with a mind-set deeply influenced by her Far Eastern roots. In her book *The Rainbow and the Worm: The Physics of Organisms*, she writes at great length about the connective tissues throughout our bodies, including muscles, tendons, and ligaments. Ho theorizes that they contain liquid crystal that facilitates communication between tissues and molecules, and in turn, enables the human body to function both effectively and coherently. In her eyes, these connective tissues are central to our health and well-being. She paints them as a link between the subtle (or imperceptible) energies on which many Eastern practices are based and the measurable energy that comprises all matter.

Dr. Ho is far from the first scientist to recognize that some or all of the major components of living organisms may be crystalline in nature—from organs, glands, and nerve

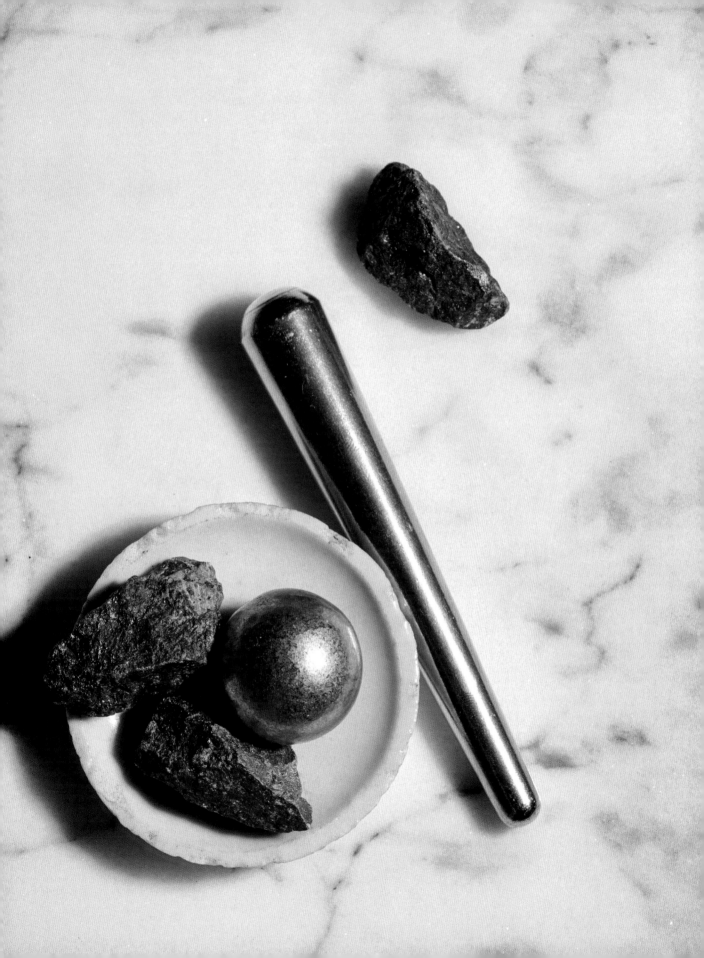

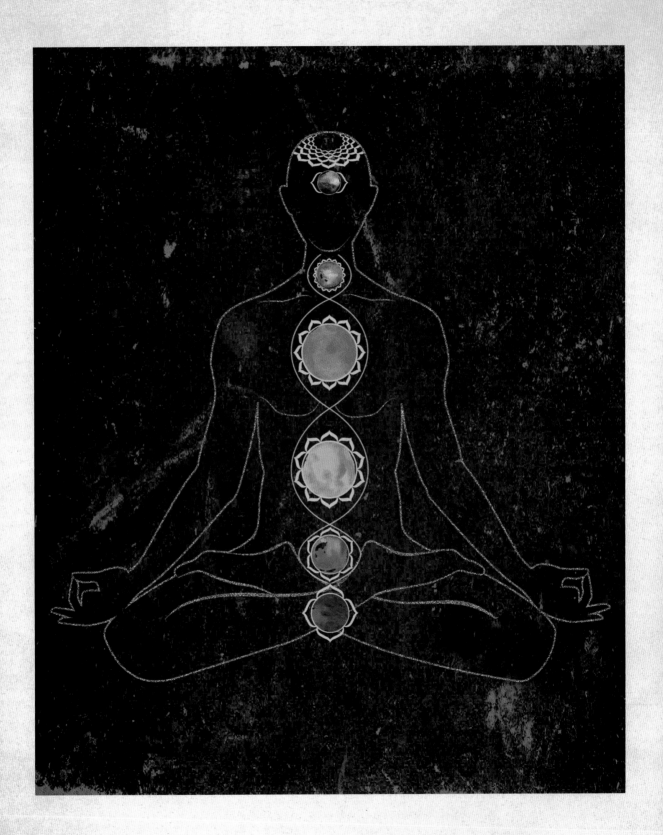

GET TO KNOW YOUR CHAKRAS

The word "chakra" is Sanskrit for "wheel" or "circle." The chakras are spinning energy centers that keep *prana* flowing through the body. The seven most widely accepted chakras start at the base of the spine (the Root chakra) and end at the crown of the head (the Crown chakra).

What they do: These points unite our physical, energetic, emotional, mental, and spiritual selves. Ideally, you want them to be balanced so that life energy flows through your body, leading you to feel healthy, vibrant, peaceful, and alert.

When they're off-kilter: Unbalanced chakras cause illness, fatigue, anxiety, and depression. Eastern medicine holds that unbalanced chakras are the root cause of many diseases and cancers. That's because each chakra is associated with a specific physical system of the body, and each chakra provides energy to a specific organ.

Ways to balance the chakras: Soaking in a warm bath or exercising are steps you can—and should—take to moderate and balance your chakras for optimal energy flow. In addition, sitting quietly, clearing your mind, and connecting to your breath for just five to ten minutes each morning can do wonders for your state of health and balance. You can also lay gemstones that correspond with various chakras on your body (see chapter 7, "Laying of Stones: Head-to-Toe Energy Flow").

systems to lipids of cellular membranes, DNA, and proteins such as collagens. But she is one of the first, in her acupuncture-related research, to introduce the theory that the meridians, or energy pathways that acupuncturists use to determine needle placement, operate through the connective tissue, due to its liquid crystalline structure.

While Becker's and Ho's theories differ, there is definite overlap between the two. After all, the electrical properties of crystals are well documented as are their unique, highly ordered structures. In their own ways, each theory serves to explain why practices that serve to balance energy require an understanding of both the human body's electrical potential and its crystalline connections.

Dr. Becker and Dr. Ho were and are especially unusual in that although they were both trained in Western medicine, each viewed and views the human body as an energy system, an attitude more grounded in the work of alternative-health practitioners like acupuncturists. A Western approach uses conventional biology, chemistry, and physics to treat the body, repairing broken parts in the human machine. It treats both physical and mental conditions the same way—with drugs designed to alter the body's chemistry.

In contrast, alternative practitioners believe in treating the entire patient in hopes of addressing the full range of physical, emotional, mental, social, spiritual, and environmental influences that affect a person's health and well-being. They do so by manipulating the *subtle energy* of the human body. This energy is described as subtle because it can't be measured using equipment that's currently at our disposal. In ayurvedic medicine, which originated in India, this energy is referred to as *prana* and flows through energy systems made up of *nadis* and chakras. In both Hindu and tantric/yogic traditions, chakras are energy points that are part of the subtle rather than the physical body. You can think of them as the portals through which energy enters and exits the body to be transformed. Chakras are the meeting points of the *nadis,* the nonphysical energy channels through which the life force, or *prana,* moves.

In Eastern medicine, subtle energy is referred to as *chi* and *qi* (Chinese) or *ki* (Japanese), and the energy system is mapped out as a network of meridians. Traditional Chinese Medicine teaches that there's a network of meridians (twenty in total) throughout the human body—in fact, you can think of them delivering energy the way blood vessels distribute blood. Twelve principal meridians help the body and its organs function. (The remaining eight meridians, known as "extraordinary meridians," are considered the energy-storage vessels of the body.) When the principal meridians are balanced and in harmony, so is your *chi,* which then flows freely throughout the body. When a meridian is imbalanced, it results in blocked *chi,* which in turn affects you physically, emotionally, and spiritually. In acupuncture and acupressure, therapists locate points along the meridians—there are more than four hundred located around the body!— and stimulate them with fine needles or pressure from the hands to balance *chi* and relieve the affected area.

American culture is slowly but surely shifting to embrace alternative medicine as a complement to Western medicine. It's increasingly common for a doctor to refer a patient to an acupuncturist, for example. When it comes to taking a holistic view of health, we're moving in the right direction. Still, even with these advances, the majority of women I know complain of feeling tired, drained, and depleted. And experts from all backgrounds have a hard time agreeing as to why.

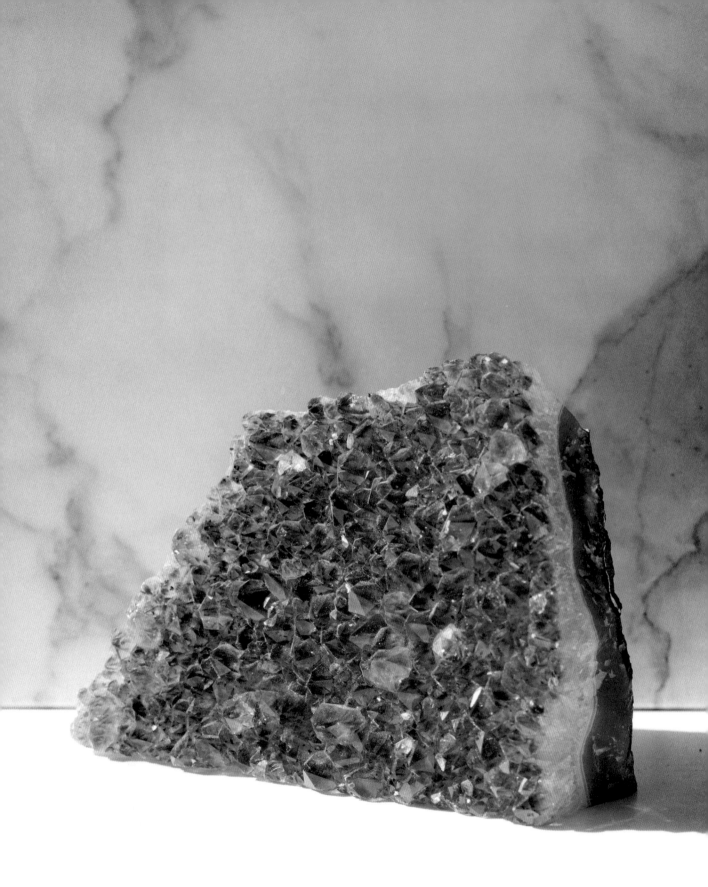

OUR ENERGY CRISIS

As I learned when I ran myself ragged in my twenties—the decade when you're supposed to have enough energy to work long hours and then socialize late into the night—there's no one answer to the question that plagues so many of us: *Why am I feeling so run-down?* When I look back now at that decade, I wonder where all my energy went. I wasn't married. I didn't have a child to raise or a business to run. I was virtually free of responsibility, with the exception of having to pay my rent and a few bills every month. Now I feel somewhat like a rubber band being pulled in various directions (and hoping I don't snap). In my ex-

> Before you buy a cell phone, find out its **specific absorption rate** (SAR). SAR is a way of measuring the quantity of radio frequency energy that is absorbed by the body. The lower the SAR of a cell phone, the better it is. Shop for a model with a SAR level of 0.5 or less.

perience, this isn't uncommon for women, or men for that matter. Just about every day a study is released that highlights some new energy-sapper, and I feel like I could be a participant in each one of those studies.

Over and over, these studies show that stress, a known precursor for depression, is the main culprit when it comes to our disappearing energy. Feeling stressed can trigger a cascade of hormones that produce physiological changes, from a rapidly beating heart and quickening of breath to tense muscles and sweaty brows or palms. Over time, repeated activation of the stress response takes a serious toll on our physical and psychological health.

Our "connected" culture and the multitasking that goes with it has only increased the stress in our daily lives, taking an even greater toll on our energy reserves. After all, in the days before smartphones, tablets, and personal computers, you rarely heard people complain about needing to "unplug"—not their electronics, but themselves. Not surprisingly, a growing body of research on multitasking suggests that while you think doing nine tasks at once increases productivity, it actually has the opposite effect. Research conducted at Stanford University in 2009 found that multitasking is in fact less productive than doing one thing at a time. Your brain can focus only on one task, so constantly switching gears means your brain needs to work a lot harder. No wonder you feel drained at the end of the day!

While we all have the ability to manage stress to some degree—by focusing on completing just one task at a time; making time to exercise; seeking out massage therapists, acupuncturists, and other practitioners to deliver a healing touch; or simply by taking a few minutes to breathe deeply in and out—there are environmental stressors as well that, without our even knowing it, deplete our energy and make us susceptible to illness. These factors can make us feel lethargic, melancholy, or just plain out of sorts.

ENVIRONMENTAL ENERGY-SAPPERS

When my husband and I moved with our son, then a toddler, into a rental house in an idyllic Connecticut suburb, I noticed the power grid a few houses away but didn't think much of it. After all, the place was temporary.

In just over a year, my symptoms started appearing: I noticed my lymph nodes swelling for no reason. Soon, they were painful and swollen every day. Then my hair started falling out. I gained six pounds out of the blue, and I started getting my period every other week. I was so exhausted that I was having trouble getting out of bed. When I consulted my acupuncturist, he thought something was wrong with my thyroid.

I did some research and learned that the thyroid is one of the first things affected when you live near a power grid. My research led me to some articles about bentonite clay detoxifying baths, which are used as therapy for cancer patients. Bentonite was used to neutralize the soil after the Chernobyl disaster. After my first bentonite clay bath, I felt like every pore in my body had been opened. I felt lighter—less lethargic and sluggish.

I also tried a tool that my mother recommended called a Tesla purple plate. She said that placing the thin aluminum rectangle under her foot when she had a broken toe had helped it heal faster. Apparently, the atomic structure of the metal is altered in such a way that it has paramagnetic properties, which aid the healing process. I placed the plates—named for Nikola Tesla, the Serbian inventor, engineer, and physicist best known for his contributions to the design of the modern alternating current (AC) electricity supply system—under my feet as well as my torso as I lay in bed at night. (It wasn't the most comfortable, but trust me, it was worth it.) I then placed several pieces of hematite, known for its pain-relief and grounding properties, by my feet, and amethyst, a stone said to promote emotional stability, strength, and healing, along major lymph nodes including blocked or amassed energy under my arms. The combination of the Tesla plates and the stones was powerful. I could feel the stagnant energy breaking up as it had during my acupuncture treatments. They also helped my lymph nodes become less swollen. When we finally moved to a new home, I continued using the plates, stones, and bentonite baths for a few more months. It took six months to get regular periods back and a year for me to feel 100 percent better.

Prior to my power-grid encounter, I had heard the term *EMF* but never quite understood what it meant. As defined by the Environmental Protection Agency, electromagnetic fields (EMFs) are a combination of electric and magnetic fields of energy, often referred to as radiation, that surround any electrical device that is plugged in and turned on. Electric fields are produced by electric charges, and magnetic fields are produced by the flow of currents through wires or electrical devices. Power lines, electrical wiring, and electrical equipment all produce EMFs. Many of the devices we come into contact with on a daily basis emit low-level radiation generally perceived as harmless to humans. Those include microwave ovens, computers, wireless (Wi-Fi) networks, cell phones, Bluetooth devices, power lines, and MRIs.

How do EMFs affect health? The official word is that there is no clear scientific evidence that they do. The International Commission on Non-Ionizing Radiation Protection has concluded that available data regarding potential long-term effects, such as increased risk of cancer, are insufficient to provide a basis for setting exposure restrictions. Still, the World Health Organization classifies electromagnetic fields as Group 2B carcinogens, which by definition means they're suspected of causing cancer. The same carcinogenic group also includes lead, engine exhaust, DDT, and chloroform.

In May 2015, a letter signed by 195 scientists from around the world called on the United Nations, the World Health Organization, and governments to develop stricter controls on devices that create EMFs. Collectively, these scientists have published more than 2,000 peer-reviewed papers on the hazards of EMFs. This letter states, "Numerous recent

YOU NEED ONLY ONE STONE TO START

In truth, all you really need to get started is one crystal in the quartz family such as amethyst, rose, citrine, or clear quartz. Clear quartz is a great universal stone to start with; because the stone has no color, it can be substituted for just about any other. It is also known to be programmable as it amplifies any energy placed into it (i.e., radio, computers, etc.) as well as other stones that you may use for a treatment, so it's a good one to have on hand no matter how small or large your collection is.

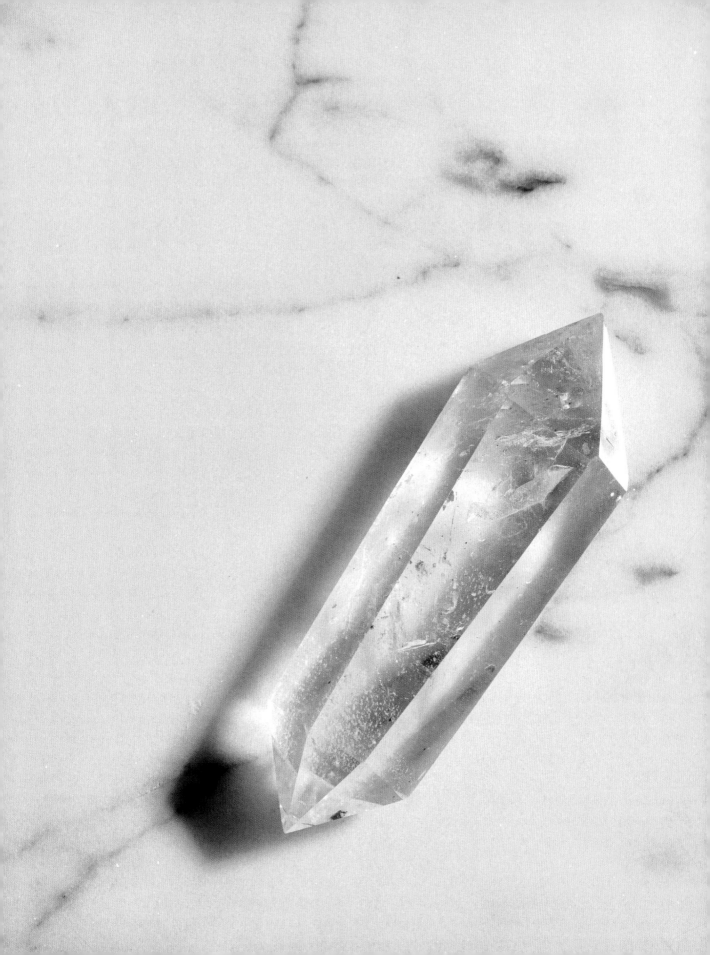

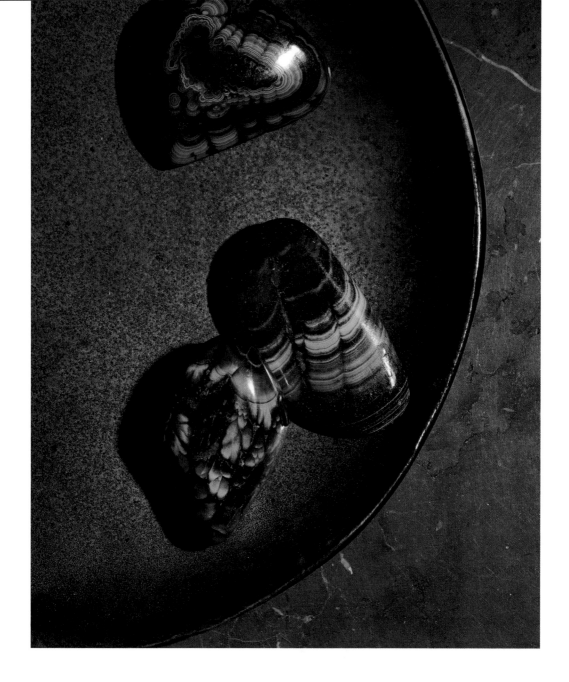

scientific publications have shown that EMF affects living organisms at levels well below most international and national guidelines. Effects include increased cancer risk, cellular stress, increase in harmful free radicals, genetic damages, structural and functional changes of the reproductive system, learning and memory deficits, neurological disorders, and negative impacts on general well-being in humans." The letter goes on to accuse the World Health Organization of failing to impose sufficient guidelines to protect the general public, particularly children, who are at greater risk.

As the mother of a young child, I am concerned. So many of the technologies that emit

Crystals and gemstones have the power—whether due to their electrical properties, unique composition and crystalline structure, or a combination thereof—to help keep your internal current (or simply, energy) flowing throughout the body.

EMFs are on or near our bodies all day long. Many of them are new enough that there hasn't been sufficient time to test their long-term effects. Governmental agencies suggest that if you're concerned about potential risks, you should reduce exposure by increasing the distance between yourself and the source. This works great if you use an earpiece rather than talking directly into your smartphone when you're on a call. But it's a little harder when the power grid is peeking through the trees in your yard. Ditto for governmental agencies' second suggestion: limit the time spent around the source. (The less time you spend near EMFs, they say, the lower your exposure.)

This advice seems a little too rudimentary, given the fact that cell-phone towers and power grids are all around us—and given our increasing dependence on smartphones, laptops, and tablets. I've been guilty of handing my son a tablet so that he can play quietly while I grocery shop or respond to a work e-mail. On one hand, these technologies are lifesavers, but I, like many moms I know, worry about the ramifications of long-term exposure to the EMFs they emit.

THE CRYSTAL / GEMSTONE BARRIER

What I've found from my extensive experimentation with crystals and gemstones is that they have the power—whether due to their electrical properties, unique composition and crystalline structure, or a combination thereof—to help keep your internal current (or simply, energy) flowing throughout the body. This, in turn, has short- and long-term benefits: In the short term, you can get through the day without feeling drained. In the long term, you build your resistance to, or, if you will, your internal barrier against, environmental threats like EMFs. What's more, the treatments in this book may help to mitigate their harsh effects after years of exposure.

All of the treatments and techniques in the pages that follow can be done at home (or on the road if you, like me, travel often). What's more, they are all steeped in tradition, whether it's the laying-of-stones ritual in chapter 7 that's been practiced for thousands of years by Hindu cultures; the Detoxifier bath in chapter 6 that uses crystals in combination with purifying clay, a tradition that dates back to ancient Mesopotamia; or the simple act of sitting with your favorite crystal in hand, setting your intention, and meditating for a few minutes every day, the oldest of all holistic rituals, dating back to at least 1500 BCE.

GET THE MOST FROM YOUR STONES

To help prepare you for what lies ahead, I want to share a little insight on what to expect and how to maximize each experience.

First, let me say that it's perfectly normal to be skeptical or apprehensive at the outset. I was, as was my mother. Looking back, I realize my apprehension had less to do with me and more to do with how I thought others would perceive the use of gemstones in our brand. Today there's talk of a crystal and gemstone "trend," but when we started our business, there was no watercooler discussion about stones' healing properties. Now here I am years later, excited to share every ounce of information I've gathered along the way from trusted vendors, chemists, physicists, and spiritual advisers. If you think about the standout moments in your life, most of them happen when you tune out the chaos in the brain and channel the true beliefs of your heart (aka your intuition). As with every new challenge, benefitting from crystal and gemstone therapies requires a willingness to transcend your current thinking while remaining open to new positive feelings and experiences.

Consistency is also important. I get it: unless you're a monk, you likely don't have countless hours to devote to any practice. The key to gaining an understanding of which gemstones resonate the most with you and which treatments and therapies are most effective is to experiment with your stones on an ongoing basis. Don't worry about having to carve out hours at a time. I've designed this book to provide a modern approach to age-old therapies. While the ancients may have had all the time in the world to explore the power of crystals and gemstones, I certainly don't. That's why I am sharing these simple treatments and techniques that I have used throughout the years, including gem elixirs, gemstone massages, gem acupressure, gem baths, and laying of stones, along with skincare and facial treatments that help you look and feel good while empowering you to ground and reconnect with the earth as well as yourself.

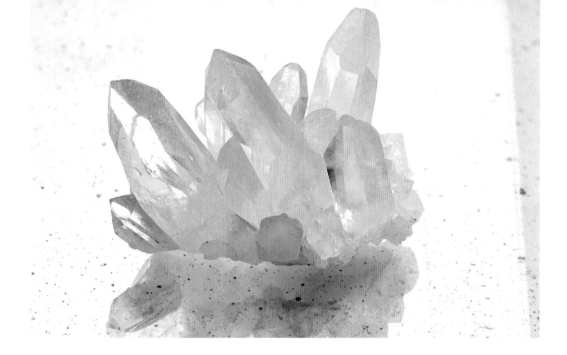

After you've tried a few, you may find yourself drawn to certain stones, and this book will help explain why. But the important thing to remember is that just as your moods change and your energy waxes and wanes, the stones that work best for these therapies and treatments may change over time as well. The good news is that there's no need to make a major investment at the outset. Chapter 3 sums up the stones and tools you'll need to get started, and you can take it from there.

Remember to give it some time. There may have been occasions when you received massages or other treatments and felt nothing on the table—and then went home and felt a sense of calm, peace, clarity, or renewal. Gem and crystal therapies work in a similar way. The results aren't often evident immediately after completing a treatment, as they tend to work on a subtle level. One way to measure change is to keep a journal in which you track how you feel an hour, a week, and a month after every treatment. Devoting a little extra time to tuning in to the incremental changes you experience will serve you well. Acquaint yourself with one crystal or gemstone at a time. Hold it, sleep with it under your pillow or on your nightstand, tote it with you, and place it on your desk while you work. Get to know it—learn about its healing history and how it affects *your* body and mind at different times of the day. If you have a pain somewhere, feel free to experiment by moving stones there to help receive their benefits. Don't just put a stone on your stomach because it's yellow. Put it where you think you need it. If you can find the place where the energy releases, you'll know it.

By slowing down and taking the time to observe your responses, you'll gain a better understanding of which gemstones and treatments resonate with you, and I can bet you'll wonder why you didn't try them sooner!

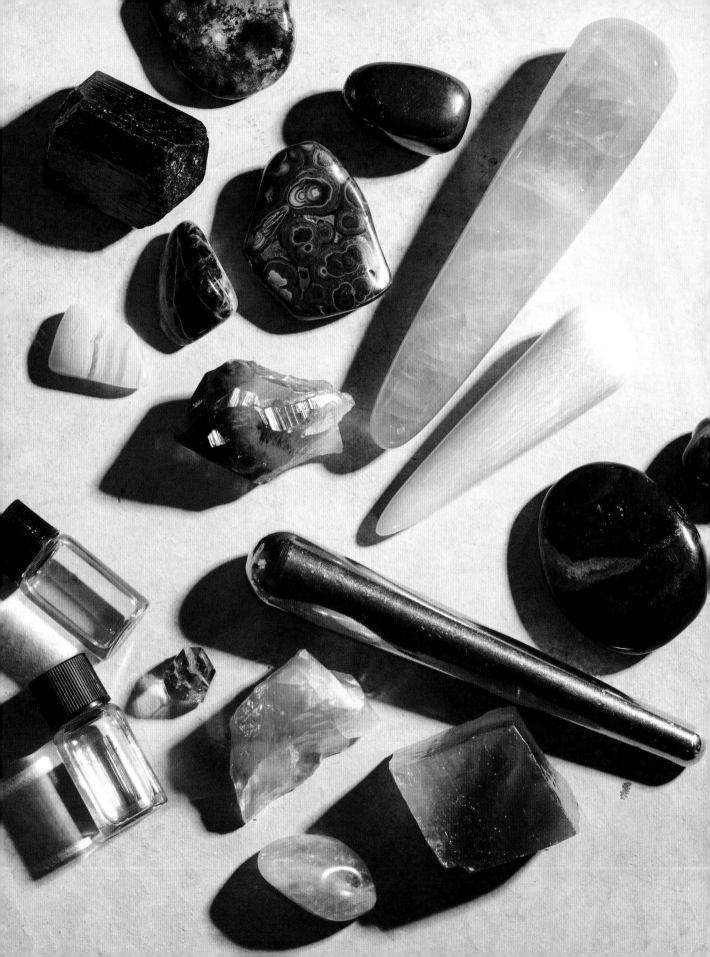

3

ESSENTIAL STONES

BUILDING YOUR COLLECTION

I'll never forget the first time I walked into Astro Gallery of Gems, a 10,000-square-foot gem and mineral showroom in New York City. After experiencing some amazing healing treatments with practitioners who used gemstones instead of acupuncture needles or hot stones to help relax my muscles and calm my nerves, I was excited to purchase my first gemstone. But the showroom space was filled with so many crystals, gems, geodes, and unusual pieces of jewelry, I felt overwhelmed. Try as I did to process all of the colors, shapes, and sparkle, my eyes didn't know where to look first.

When I told the salesperson what properties I was interested in, he led me to a glass case containing dozens of smaller specimens in shades of pink, green, purple, blue, and metallic black. Some were smooth and round; others were jagged with distinct crystalline faces. But their soothing colors immediately calmed me.

Until that day I had no idea just how many crystals and gemstones exist in the world. Not even mineral experts can pinpoint the exact figure, which is estimated at somewhere between two thousand and four thousand, and more are discovered every year. It's virtually impossible to record every mineral found because even the tiniest variation in heat or pressure or the introduction of impurities can determine which crystal or gemstone will form as a result. The combinations seem (and are) virtually endless. I honestly don't know how gemologists and mineralogists keep them all straight!

Since I'd already done some research for my business, I was familiar with a handful of stones like rose quartz, amethyst, and jade. But I'd never before heard of or seen some of the spectacular stones in that case, from dark blue azurite and transparent cherry sphalerite to translucent green vivianite. Each time the knowledgeable salesman, John, mentioned the origin of a particular stone—from India to Morocco to China—I felt as if he'd added another stamp to my passport.

I walked out of the store that day not only with a rose quartz from Brazil, but also with a much greater appreciation for the mineral world—and a fantastic recommendation for a crystal and gemstone practitioner: John's aunt, Camille. Camille has since become an invaluable resource for helping me to understand the various therapeutic uses for stones.

LITTLE GEM

While the majority of crystals and gemstones are inorganic, meaning they come from rock or other nonliving materials, there are a small number of organic gemstones that bear little resemblance to the sparklers you might associate with decorative gems. Among them are pearl, coral, and amber.

As gemstones have evolved from the cornerstone of the skincare line that my mother and I cofounded to a personal passion, my collection has continued to expand. The stones in our possession range from tiny chips we use for product testing to oversize decorative geodes. (Of course, with a rambunctious five-year-old, I've moved the majority of my more valuable stones to the office until he's a little older.) In between the chips and geodes, there are hundreds of tumbled stones and dozens of crystal and gemstone wands, which are perfect for massage and reflexology treatments. Trust me—with a five-year-old at home, I use them. A lot!

These days, between my mother's personal collection and my own, we're giving Astro Gallery of Gems a run for their money! Among the stones we've found while traveling around the United States, China, South America, Thailand, and Indonesia are blue sapphire, malachite, citrine, fluorite, carnelian, scolecite, apophyllite, aquamarine, aqua and yellow obsidian, and celestine. My mother and I use stones to calm us when we travel and to clear the energy in hotel rooms (see "Stones for Travel," page 205, for more tips), and we also both use business and personal trips as an opportunity to collect unusual specimens. Recent acquisitions include three beautiful blue copper stones Mom found when in Denver for a family wedding, and a lovely small but clear amethyst from Iguazu Falls in Brazil.

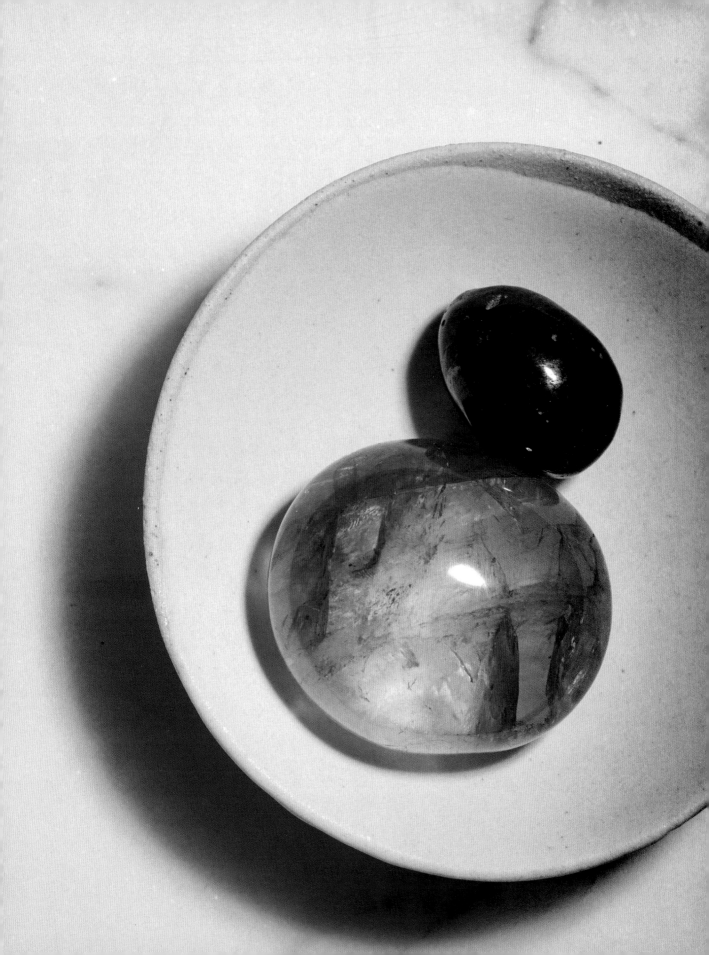

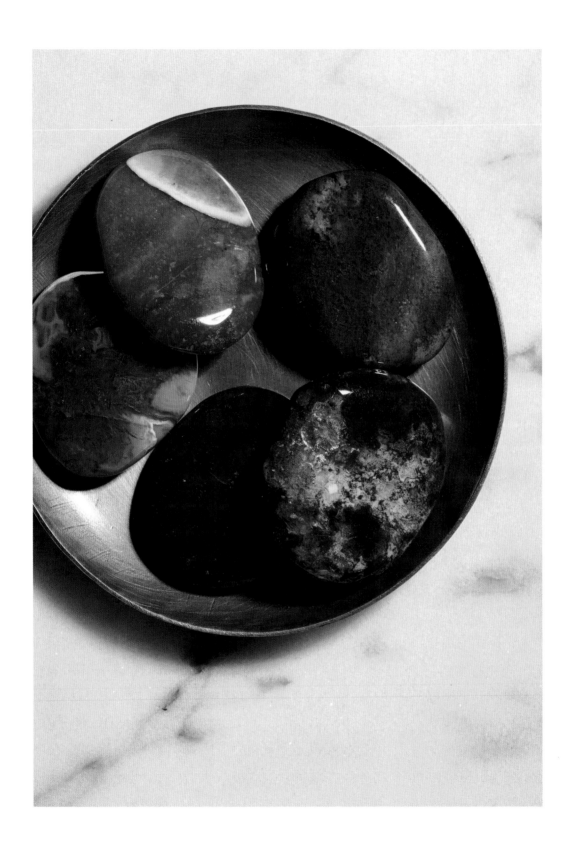

Collecting crystals and gemstones has become a bit of an obsession for us in part because each stone has such an interesting story to tell. But the last thing I want for *you* to feel is overwhelmed by the array of choices available—or to worry about buying the "right" stones or about having enough stones to truly experience their therapeutic benefits. You definitely don't need an extensive collection to experience all that crystals and gemstones have to offer. To get you started on your personal gemstone journey, I've selected ten stones of various hues that compose a fantastic, multitasking collection. They're by no means the only stones you'll ever need, but they will suffice until you decide you want to expand your collection. If you're lucky enough to live someplace where there are retailers that sell quality crystals and gems, I highly suggest buying them in person; they're a lot like potential

ASK YOURSELF BEFORE YOU BUY

How do you narrow your search when there are so many compelling stones? Answering the questions below before you shop will help keep you focused. I do suggest that you allow yourself a certain degree of latitude, however, should you be drawn to a stone that is different from the one you had initially envisioned. This is very different from acting on impulse. Spend a little time with the stone. Hold it in your hand. Do you feel a slight "magnetic pull" or pulsations? Does it feel right, visually, intuitively, and physically? If you're not sure, put the stone back and wait a bit. Believe me, if that stone is meant to go home with you, it will!

What stones are you attracted to?

What are your favorite colors?

Do you prefer pale or deep shades?

Do you prefer tumbled stones, cut faceted stones, or raw stones?
This will depend on whether you prefer the look of polished stones or those that are completely natural. Polished and tumbled stones have a soft, harmonizing effect, while unpolished or cut stones are powerful and invigorating.

What will you be using the stone for? Self-care rituals like massage? Creating elixirs? Bathing? Meditation? Decoration? Jewelry?

How much are you prepared to spend?

partners—you never really know if there's chemistry until you actually meet. If that's not an option, I've worked with many trustworthy online retailers over the years, whose information is listed in the resource guide beginning on page 215.

Whichever gemstone or crystal you're purchasing, there are a few things to keep in mind when you set out to shop for one. First, you want to make sure you're getting the stone you think you're getting. If you're prepared to spend a lot of money on a precious stone, it should come with a GIA (Gemological Institute of America) appraisal certification. If you have any doubts about the stone being real, take it to a gemologist and have it checked.

Semiprecious stones, such as amethyst, topaz, or turquoise, for example, are a little trickier. There are a lot of imitation and synthetic semiprecious stones out there, which are easy to mistake for the real deal. Imitation stones are either glass or plastic, both of which materials lack the crystalline structure and natural origins and life force that make them effective tools for healing and meditation. Generally, if a stone is super-clear or extremely sparkly, lacks any nicks or scratches, *and* is very affordable, it is likely not a real gemstone or crystal. Another thing to look out for is synthetic crystals. While they have the same composition and nearly identical optical and physical properties as real ones, synthetics can be tough to spot without advanced instrumentation. A rule of thumb that I follow, whether shopping at a tried-and-true store or someplace I've never been before, is if you're holding a natural quartz and a synthetic version, the natural quartz will remain cold for longer than the synthetic one does, because natural stones have a higher thermal conductivity than glass. On an interesting note, synthetics can be charged with the natural stone of the same origin when using a copper pyramid.

You may also come across crystals and gems that are treated to deepen their color (e.g., aquamarine, smoky quartz, and citrine). But don't worry: as long as the stone is natural, it is suitable for therapeutic treatments and techniques.

THE ELEMENTAL TEN

YOUR CRYSTAL AND GEMSTONE STARTER KIT

My list of ten essential crystals and gems is the result of many conversations with Camille, who's been collecting stones and using their healing power on clients for more than three decades, as well as my own independent trial-and-error research. I chose these stones for various reasons, the most important being color, safety, and skin and soul benefits.

COLOR

The hues of gemstones and crystals take on new meaning when used for therapeutic treatments. I've devoted chapter 7 of this book to the same chakra-balancing treatments that were written more than five thousand years ago in ancient Vedic texts, so I wanted to make sure you have access to the colors that correspond with the various energy centers along the body, allowing you to experience their healing benefits from feet to forehead and beyond. If you can't get your hands on one or more of the stones on the following pages, just aim to find another from the same color group. I've suggested several alternatives for every stone, but there are even more that you can try, as long as they're similarly hued.

SAFETY

When making elixirs or bathing, be sure to use stones that are nontoxic, as well as those that are not water-soluable. Quartz is normally a safe bet.

GOOD FOR SKIN AND SOUL

Based on what I've learned over more than a dozen years of testing själ prototypes on all skin types, I wanted to recommend stones that are complementary for the skin. And since the Swedish name we chose for our business, själ, literally translates to "spirit, mind, heart, and soul," the ability of stones to transport you spiritually was also important. I chose blue sapphire, for example, because of its age-old ability to connect the mind and the body with the spirit and soul. (That's also the main reason I've used Himalayan sapphire elixir in my product line since 2001.)

I encourage you to start slowly. In your left hand, hold a particular stone you find interesting (due to its color, shape, or texture) for at least 20 minutes every day the first week. The next week, try one treatment or technique and pay close attention to how you feel afterward. Remember, every stone is unique, and sometimes the very same stone can affect individuals differently. Clear quartz, for instance, raises my energy level to a point at which I am energized and ready to take on any big projects I've been avoiding. When my husband holds the same clear quartz stone, he's almost too energetic. For him, milder rose quartz or smoky quartz are great alternatives.

Once you've sampled a few of the treatments and techniques in the chapters that follow, you'll likely find that you connect to a particular stone or stones, and you can then begin expanding your collection by finding others in the same color family or with similar properties. Start slowly and graduate to your comfort level.

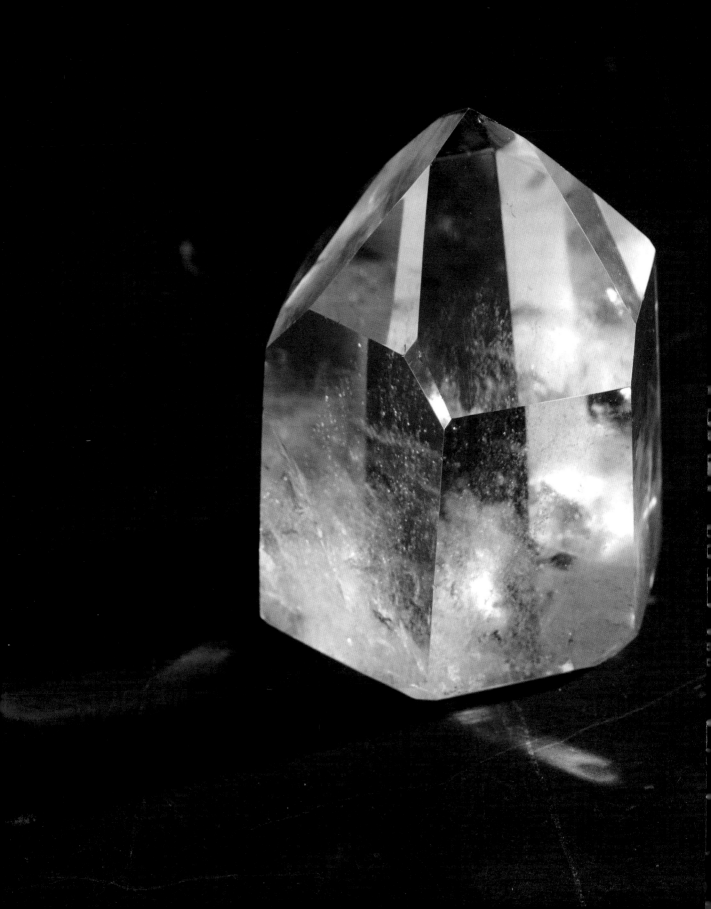

CLEAR QUARTZ

ESSENTIAL FOR BALANCE, FOCUS, AND CLARITY

Also known as crystal quartz or rock crystal, this versatile "white light" is the single most important stone to have on hand. Its colorlessness means you can substitute it for any stone in any treatment or practice. You can also use this high-vibrational stone to amplify the energy of other stones in baths, elixirs, or face and body treatments.

Color: Colorless

Found in: Canada, Brazil, Germany, Madagascar, China, South Africa, Venezuela, and the United States

Mind/body benefits: Aids in spiritual growth, brings balance, and promotes and restores well-being

Healing properties: Known to stimulate the immune system; believed to help dissipate blockages and promote energy flow, thereby boosting the brain and nervous system

Corresponding chakras: All, but particularly the Crown

History and legend: In ancient times, clear quartz was thought to be a form of nonmelting ice. In fact, the word "crystal" comes from *krustallos*, the Greek word for "ice." That may explain why it was once believed to quench thirst.

Alternative clear stones: Herkimer diamond, diamond, and colorless danburite

Due to its ability to amplify, clear quartz should be used in a positive mode or to make other crystals work in harmony.

AMETHYST

ESSENTIAL FOR CLEANSING AND PURIFYING

Fine amethysts have long been fixtures in religious jewelry and royal crown jewels. They were once considered equal in value to rubies, emeralds, and sapphires, but over time became more readily available and, hence, less "precious." Amethysts still adorn the fingers of the pope, as well as the coronation regalia of British royalty. Their purple hue, much like that of the highest chakra (the Crown), is known to enhance intuition and connect one with the energy of heaven and spiritual freedom.

Color: Pale lavender to deep violet

Found in: Brazil, Canada, Russia, Uruguay, South Korea, and the United States

Mind/body benefits: Known as "nature's tranquilizer," the stone promotes awareness, peacefulness, and contentment; wards off negativity and nightmares; and helps to heal during times of personal loss, grief, and sadness

Healing properties: Believed to relieve tension headaches and eye strain and soothe itching and other skin irritations; believed to help with addiction

Corresponding chakras: Third Eye and Crown

History and legend: Ancient Greeks and Romans drank wine from goblets of carved amethyst because it was believed to prevent and cure drunkenness.

Alternative purple stones: Purple tourmaline, iolite, sugilite, and charoite

Moistening an amethyst and rubbing it over blemishes helps to calm irritation.

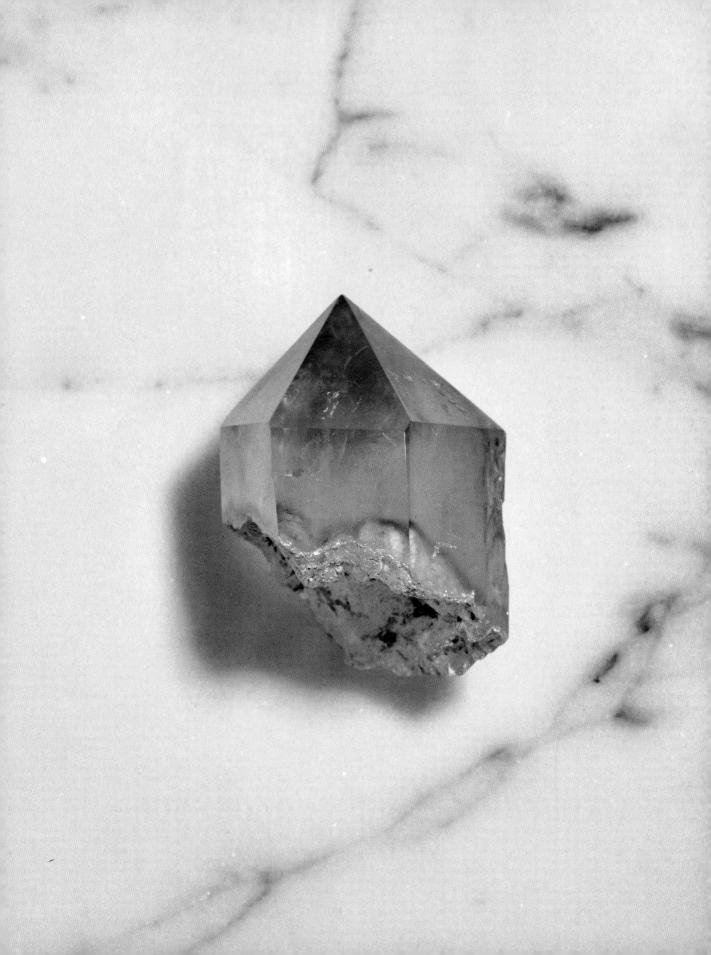

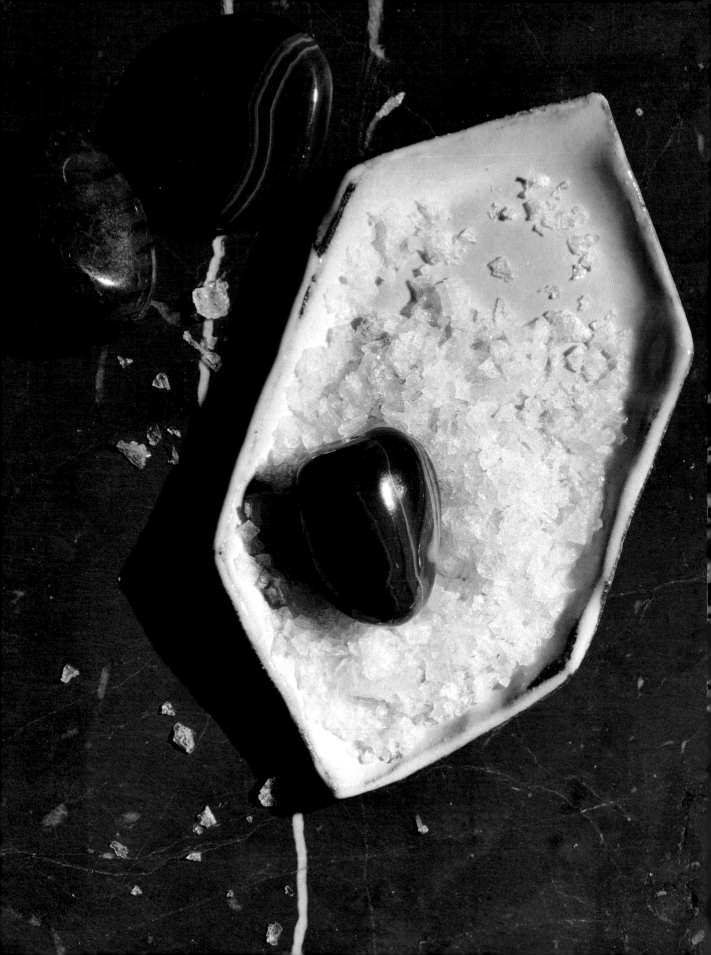

CARNELIAN

ESSENTIAL FOR STRENGTHENING AND STIMULATING

Carnelian has long been thought to bring good luck to its wearer. Considered a stone of kings, carnelian is said to promote courage and provide protection. It was worn extensively in ancient Egypt to avert the powers of the Evil Eye and to bring peace to the wearer. Later, in Europe, Napoleon wore a carnelian ring with a similar seal to keep him safe in battle.

Color: Red-orange to brownish-red

Found in: India, Brazil, Uruguay, and the United States

Mind/body benefits: Increases ambition, drive, confidence, and creativity; dispels boredom, apathy, and passivity

Healing properties: Believed to help with digestive issues and reduce pain associated with the abdomen and menstrual and menopausal symptoms; may also be beneficial for childbirth and boosting physical energy

Corresponding chakra: Sacral (second)

History and legend: Carnelian is one of the stones people have been cutting and polishing the longest in recorded human history. Its use dates back more than four thousand years. According to the Old Testament, it was one of the twelve gemstones worn on the breastplate of Aaron, the first high priest of the Israelites and a prophet.

Alternative orange stones: Fire opal, orange sunstone, orange garnet (spessartine), orange calcite, and tangerine quartz

Meditating with carnelian helps increase drive and ambition, which makes it the perfect stone to assist with career-related decisions.

CITRINE

ESSENTIAL FOR MENTAL CLARITY, OPTIMISM, AND REGENERATION

Often called "lemon quartz," this stone's name is derived from the Latin word for yellow. Due to its color, citrine was once prescribed as a cure for jaundice and other diseases of the liver, but it has since become associated with new pursuits and sunny dispositions.

Color: Yellow-brown

Found in: Brazil, Russia, and Madagascar

Mind/body benefits: Enhances mental clarity, confidence, willpower, and personal power; encourages openness; stabilizes emotions; and calms anger and frustration

Healing properties: Known to be beneficial for digestive and toxicity issues; may also relieve symptoms such as depression, self-doubt, and anger

Corresponding chakra: Solar Plexus

History and legend: In ancient times, citrine was thought to offer protection from both snake venom and evil thoughts. Citrine, long referred to as a "success stone" or "merchant's stone," is also thought to increase wealth if carried with you or kept in your home.

Alternative yellow stones: Amber, yellow jade, yellow sunstone, and yellow beryl

Citrine is said to manifest abundance, success, and good fortune.

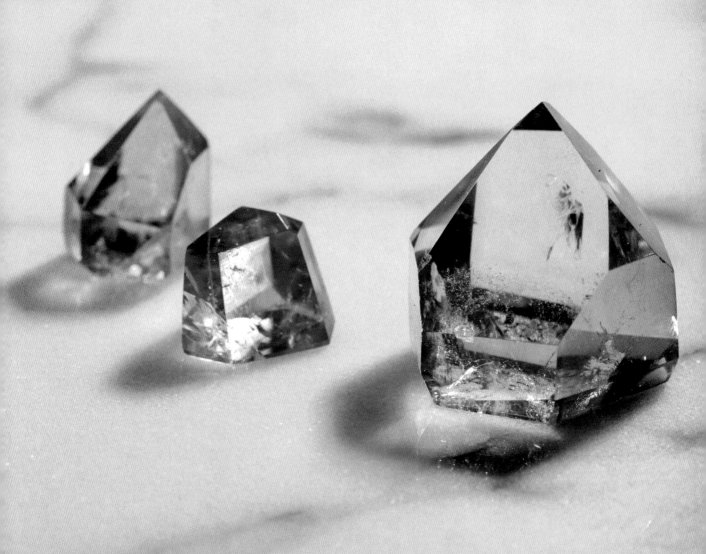

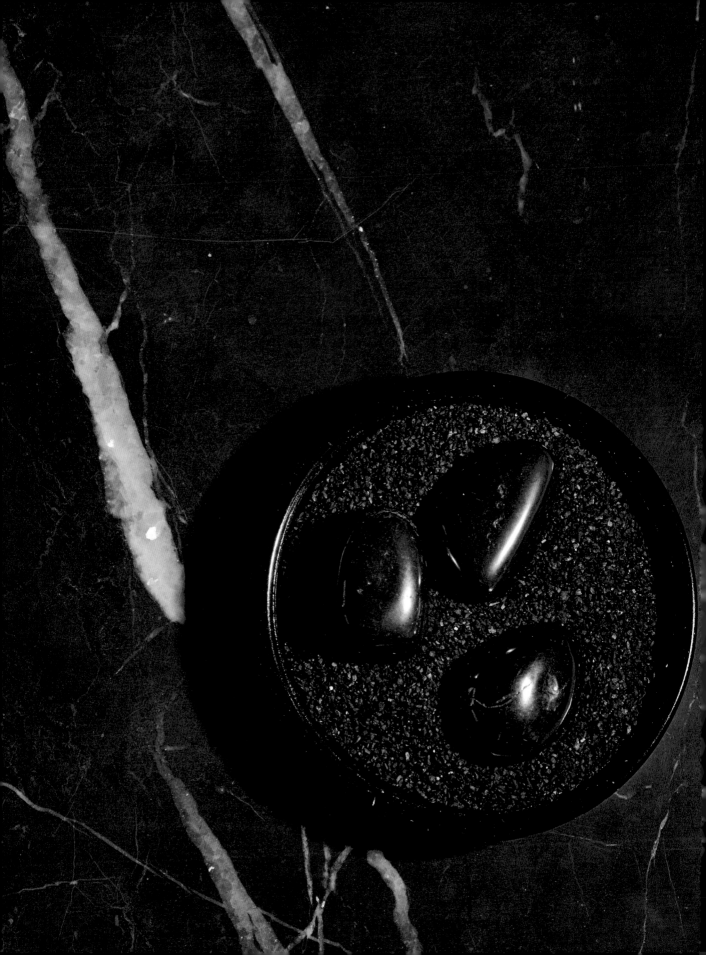

HEMATITE

ESSENTIAL FOR ENERGIZING WHILE ALSO GROUNDING

This common stone found in sedimentary, metamorphic, and igneous rocks will keep your mind from wandering and your feet firmly planted. It is the primary ore used to make iron and also has oxygenating properties, great for energizing and de-puffying the skin and eye area.

Color: Black to steel- or silver-gray, brown to reddish-brown, or red

Found in: Canada, Australia, Mexico, South America, Africa, Europe, Asia, Greenland, England, Brazil, and the United States

Mind/body benefits: Grounds, stabilizes, energizes, and protects; helps to balance meridians and provide equilibrium to mind, body, and spirit; enhances thought, memory, and concentration; and can also prevent you from feeling spacey or overwhelmed

Healing properties: Thought to have a strengthening effect in cases of fatigue and weakness; may also promote the uptake of iron in the body, stimulate circulation, and improve wound healing

Corresponding chakra: Root (Base)

History and legend: The stone gets its name from the Greek word for "blood," perhaps because it turns deep red when ground into powder. Ancient Romans used the powder as war paint in hopes that it would make them invincible (and possibly invisible) during battles.

Alternative dark stones: Black tourmaline, obsidian, and smoky quartz

Polished hematite stones were once used as mirrors. Today, the protective stone is believed to work somewhat like a boomerang to mirror energy and send it back to the originator.

GREEN MOSS AGATE

ESSENTIAL FOR CONFIDENCE BOOSTING AND PERSONAL GROWTH

This stone is said to bring abundance, success, and prosperity to both farmers and gardeners and to others who recognize its powers. Known as the agate of warriors, moss agate is considered the most powerful of the agates.

Color: Green, often with brown and red patterns

Found in: Brazil, Argentina, Uruguay, Mexico, Poland, India, Australia, and the United States

Mind/body benefits: Balances emotions as well as enhancing concentration, persistence, endurance, and success

Healing properties: Thought to help improve circulation and enhance healing of all types; may also support the lymphatic and immune system and help ease kidney, bladder, and pancreatic issues; believed to help enhance oxygen in the body

Corresponding chakras: Heart and Third Eye

History and legend: Agate is said to have been discovered sometime around the third or fourth century BCE by Theophrastus, a Greek philosopher, who named the stone after the river in which it was found. Green moss agate is aptly named, since its color resembles moss or trees and represents new growth, either personal or spiritual.

Alternative green stones: Green jasper, green jadeite, green tourmaline, aventurine, emerald, jade, and malachite

Moss agate is sometimes called the "birthing crystal" because it's said to ease childbirth.

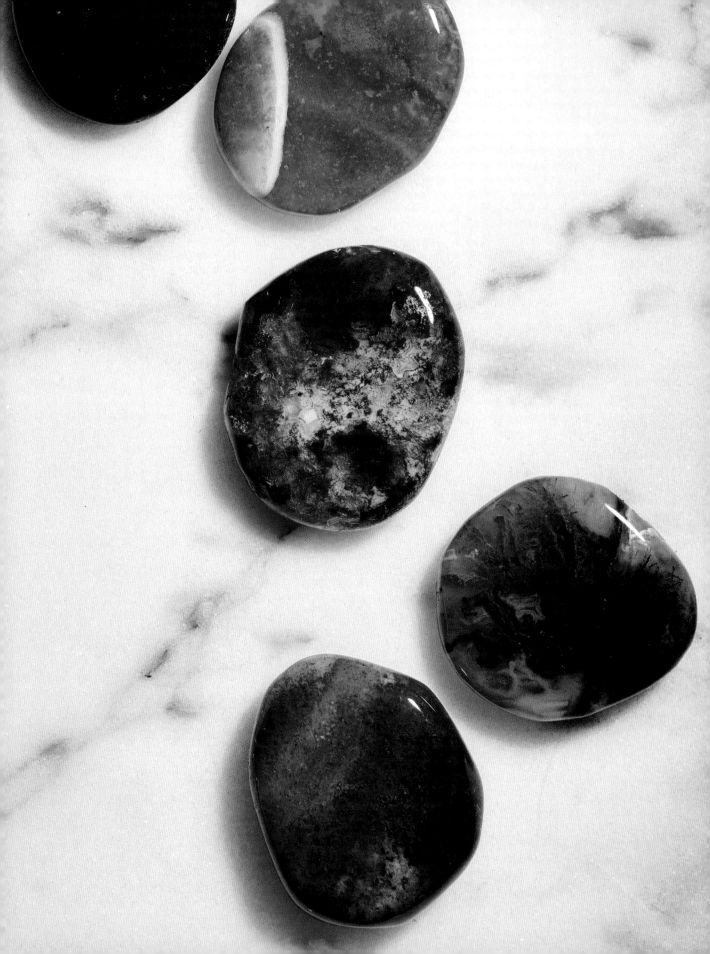

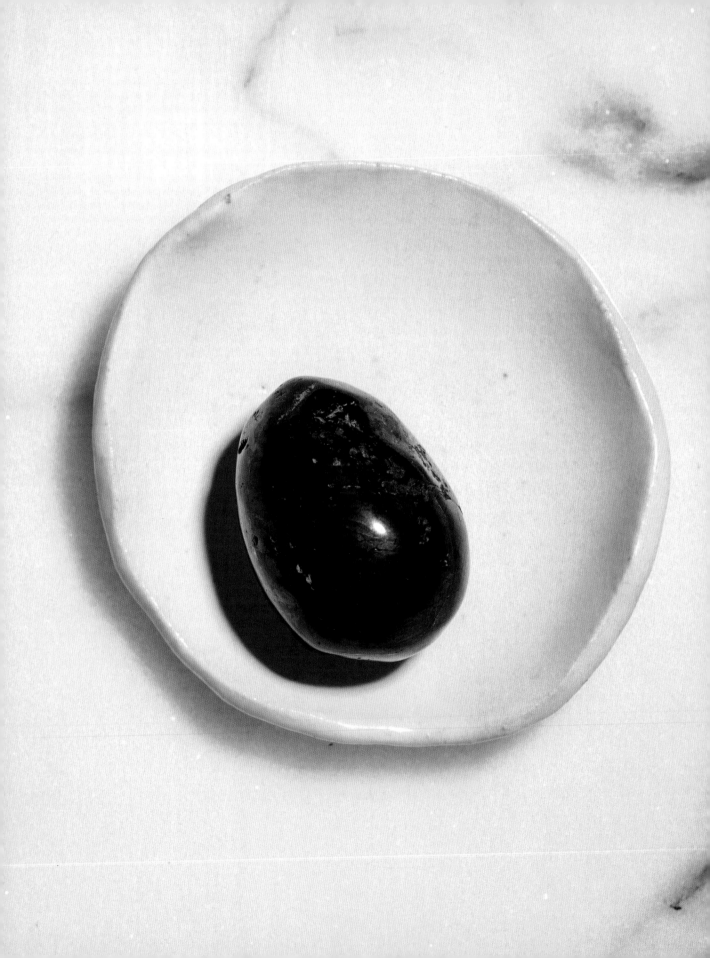

RED JASPER

ESSENTIAL FOR WARMING AND STABILIZING

Red jasper was held in high esteem by ancient Babylonians and Egyptians, who associated it with the blood of life and often carved it into protective amulets used to protect the heart. A microcrystalline variety of quartz and a member of the chalcedony family, it often contains organic material and iron oxides that account for its interesting patterns and bands.

Color: Red, sometimes spotted, ringed, or striped

Found in: Australia, Brazil, Canada, Egypt, India, Indonesia, Kazakhstan, Madagascar, Mexico, Russia, Uruguay, Venezuela, and the United States

Mind/body benefits: Known as a spiritually grounding stone; helps to strengthen and balance; also believed to enhance perseverance, stamina, endurance, and creative passion, and helps to alleviate anger issues

Healing properties: Thought to boost circulation and blood flow

Corresponding chakras: Base and Sacral

History and legend: Red jasper symbolizes the blood of the earth in many Native American cultures and is thought to help connect its wearers with the stabilizing energies of the earth. Throughout time, it has also been used to protect against evil spirits and to bring courage and relief from pain.

Alternative red stones: Ruby, red spinel, red garnet, cuprite, red agate, and red quartz

Looking to heat things up in the bedroom? Like all red stones, red jasper signifies passion, and it's known to promote sexual compatibility and enhance sex.

ROSE QUARTZ

ESSENTIAL FOR NURTURING AND HEALING

Don't let its gentle pastel hue fool you. This stone is a powerhouse, subtly soothing body and mind and opening the heart to new experiences. Though rose quartz is often too cloudy to be cut into gemstones, the occasional clear stone is cut and polished for decorative use.

Color: Pale pink to red rose

Found in: Brazil

Mind/body benefits: Grounds, soothes, nurtures, helps to manifest unconditional love and forgiveness, and promotes sensitivity; also helps to alleviate fears while promoting a sense of security

Healing properties: Known to stabilize blood circulation and improve blood flow; believed to help support the kidneys and lungs and promote fertility; also helps calm red complexion

Corresponding chakras: Heart, Solar Plexus, and Sacral

History and legend: Dating back to 7000 BCE, the stone was initially mined in Mesopotamia (now Iraq). Ancient Romans, Egyptians, and Greeks used it as a talisman. The Egyptians also believed it could prevent aging.

Alternative pink stones: Pink or watermelon tourmaline, morganite, pink apatite, pink quartz, pink garnet, and rhondonchriste

Small amounts of the element titanium give rose quartz its color.

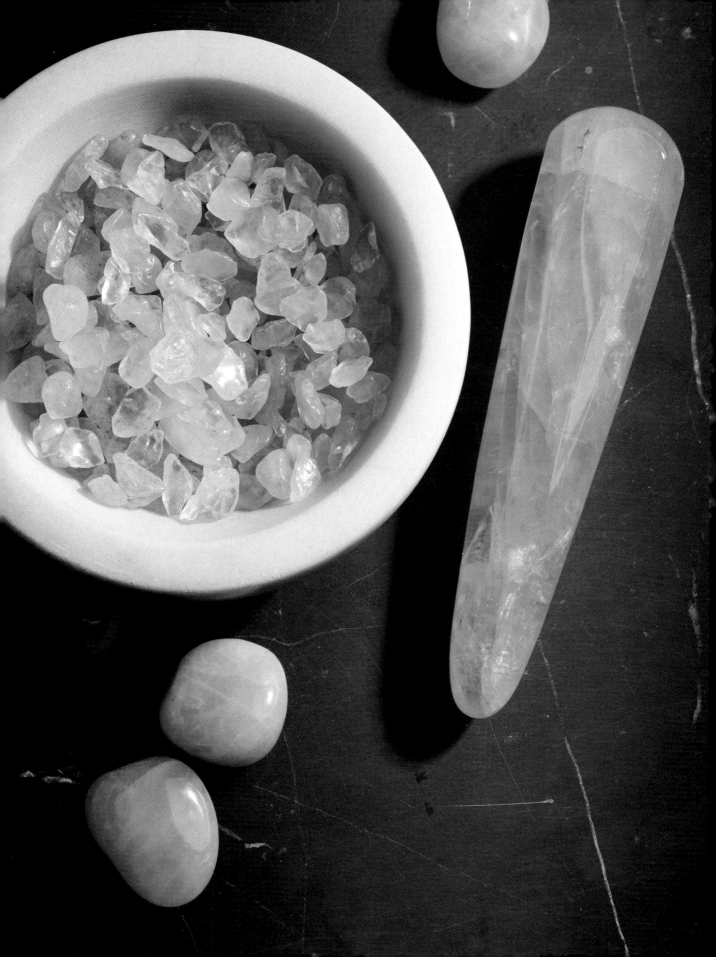

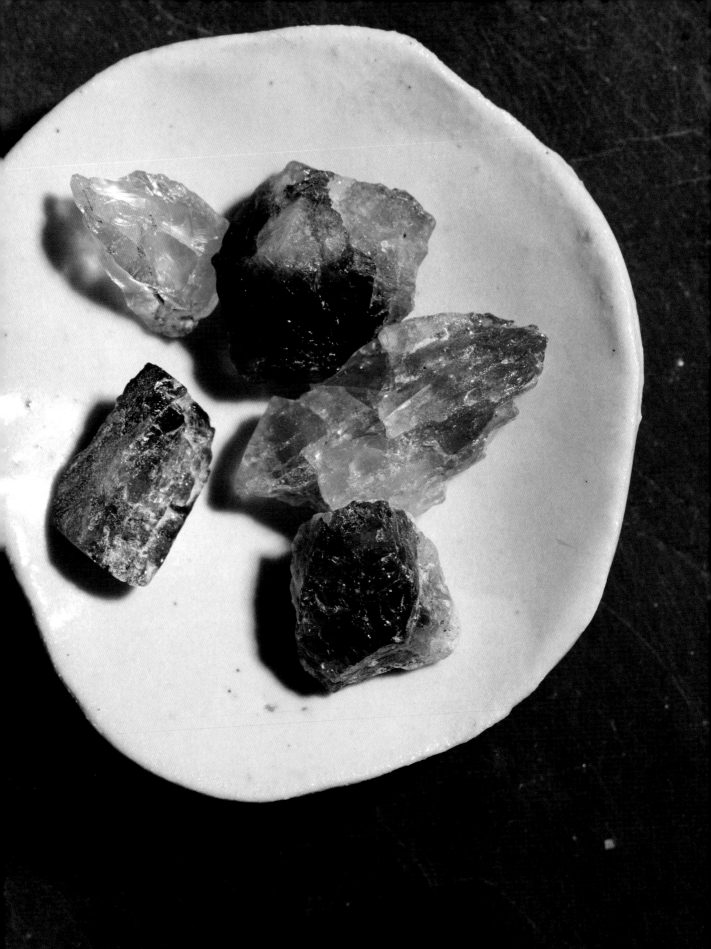

SAPPHIRE

ESSENTIAL FOR CLEARING, CONNECTING TO THE SPIRIT, AND DEVOTION

Sapphires have been prized since antiquity. In fact, some of the very first gems ever to be cut and polished were sapphires. According to Eastern tradition, the sapphire is thought to connect the mind and the body by stimulating the pituitary gland (which helps produce melatonin), thereby relaxing the body.

Color: Cornflower blue

Found in: Australia, Malawi, Madagascar, Sri Lanka, and the United States

Mind/body benefits: Promotes learning and wisdom as well as mental acuity

Healing properties: Known to aid hormonal glands (pituitary and hypothalamus) and digestive organs

Corresponding chakras: Throat, Third Eye, Solar Plexus, and Heart

History and legend: To the ancient and medieval world, the gem's heavenly blue signified the height of celestial hope and faith. Sapphires were thought to protect their wearers from evil. In the Middle Ages, Europeans believed that sapphires cured eye diseases and preserved chastity. Deep blue sapphires, long associated with royalty, were often worn by medieval kings who believed that the gemstones would protect them from their enemies. Up until the late seventeenth century, sapphires were reserved for royalty, nobility, and high-ranking clergy in England—anyone else caught wearing them would be punished. The stones have since become symbolic of nobility, divinity, and faithfulness.

Alternative blue stones: Blue lace agate, lapis, sodalite, turquoise, aquamarine, larimar, and azurite

Sapphires are believed to significantly improve your problem-solving ability by inspiring clarity of vision and thought.

SCOLECITE

ESSENTIAL FOR CALMING AND AWAKENING THE HEART

This peaceful stone helps to promote a very relaxed and uplifted feeling, which makes it wonderful to use in meditation. It is said to be especially beneficial to those who suffer from panic attacks.

Color: Milky white or colorless

Found in: India, Iceland, Scotland, Brazil, Russia, and the United States

Mind/body benefits: Facilitates deep inner peace and spiritual transformation, helping you take control of your life

Healing properties: Known to promote circulation; may help with insomnia; also good for massage and relaxing skin

Corresponding chakras: Heart, Third Eye, and Crown

History and legend: The ancients likely never encountered scolecite, which was first recognized as a mineral species in 1813 in Germany and named ten years later. The name comes from the German *skolezit,* which stems from the Greek word for "worm," alluding to the fact that the crystals often curl when heated.

Alternative white stones: Milky quartz, white marble, moonstone, and selenite

Having trouble sleeping? Scolecite is your stone, since it is said to enhance the dream state and facilitate dream recall as well as promote restful slumber.

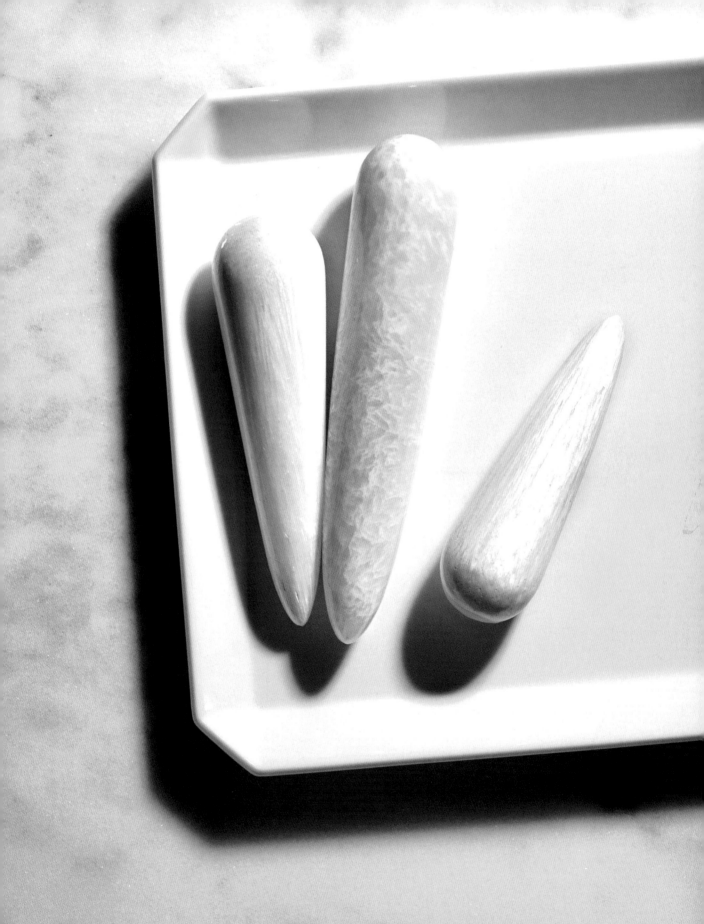

GROUNDING AND ENERGIZING STONES

When you learn to listen to your body by experimenting with the treatments and therapies in subsequent chapters, you'll begin to better understand what's throwing it out of whack. Some days you may need a little lift, while other days you may feel a little "out there" and need to be brought back down to earth. That's where stones come in. Some have grounding properties, while others are known to boost energy. As a rule of thumb, blue and purple stones are for calming, communication, and divine connection. Green are for healing, dark stones are for grounding, and red and orange stones are for warming and energizing. Here are some of each that you may want to consider adding to your healing arsenal as you grow your personal collection:

GROUNDING

These stones are best known for their stabilizing properties.

Black tourmaline

Known as a powerful grounding stone that possesses an electrical charge, black tourmaline is associated with health and protection. It is believed to help connect the human spirit with the earth.

Smoky quartz

This stone is known for centering, grounding, and removing negative energy. Smoky quartz works on the lower three chakras (Root/Base, Sacral, and Solar Plexus).

Malachite

A rich green-colored stone used for grounding, strengthening, and emotional healing, malachite is known to protect against electromagnetic pollutants and radiation.

Black obsidian

A protective stone made from volcanic glass, obsidian is thought to be excellent for psychic protection and helping to remove negativity and imbalances.

ENERGIZING

These stones are nature's answer to caffeinated beverages.

Ruby

This red stone is believed to boost stamina, and it provides renewed energy and helps to overcome exhaustion. (Raw, uncut rubies are much less expensive and are perfect for this type of healing.)

Hematite

An energizing and grounding stone, hematite is known for strengthening, vitality, and mind-body balance.

Carnelian

This vibrant stone is known for boosting energy levels and is great for creativity, vitality, drive, and determination.

Red jasper

A stone known to strengthen energy, increase life force, and provide a sense of stability and balance, red jasper is used to help stabilize aura and raise kundalini.

BRINGING HOME
YOUR CRYSTALS AND GEMS

When you purchase a stone, there's no way of knowing who has come into contact with it and whether that person's energy was positive or negative. So before you use the stone for any treatment or technique, you'll want to clean and charge it. By doing both, you're basically erasing others' energy. You'll want to clean your stone each time you use it. But don't ever use soap! Instead, try one of two methods: wet or dry.

All of the stones recommended in this chapter can be cleaned using the wet or dry method; the wet method entails leaving them to soak in salt water. Simply fill a glass or ceramic bowl (not metal, which could cause a chemical reaction with certain stones) about half full and place your stones in the salt water so that they are fully submerged. Let them rest for anywhere between one and twenty-four hours. Then thoroughly rinse the stones in cool running water to remove any remaining salt. One caveat: Stones that should not be soaked in salt water include crystals that are porous, contain metal, or have a water content, such as opal, selenite, calcite, and fluorite (see "Hold the Water," page 80). As a rule, you should avoid water cleansing with crystals that are below Mohs' (hardness) scale of three, a measurement you can usually find online. If you aren't sure of your crystal's Mohs' rating, then avoid water cleansing to be on the safe side.

> **LITTLE GEM**
>
> Placing your entire crystal collection in one bowl—known as "crystal crowding"—can sap the stones' energy. Plus, it makes them more difficult to admire and appreciate. Instead, try grouping stones of like colors (four or five each) on your desk, nightstand, or bookshelf. Alternatively, you can enhance the stones using clear crystal quartz.

Stones that can't be soaked or you are unsure of should be cleaned with running water or the dry method, which entails immersing them directly in sea salt. Fill a glass bowl halfway up with sea salt and either bury your stones in the dry salt or leave them on its surface, depending on the amount of negative-energy clearing the stone may require. Stones should be left in or on the salt for anywhere from several hours to several days. Remove any remaining salt with a soft, dry cloth. Always throw away the salt after use.

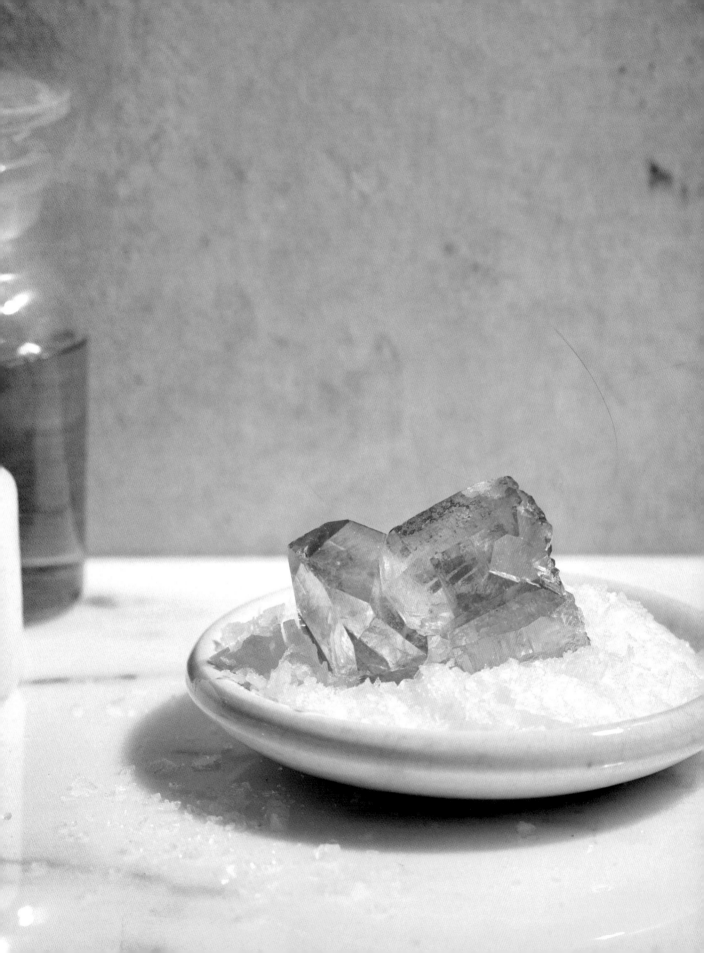

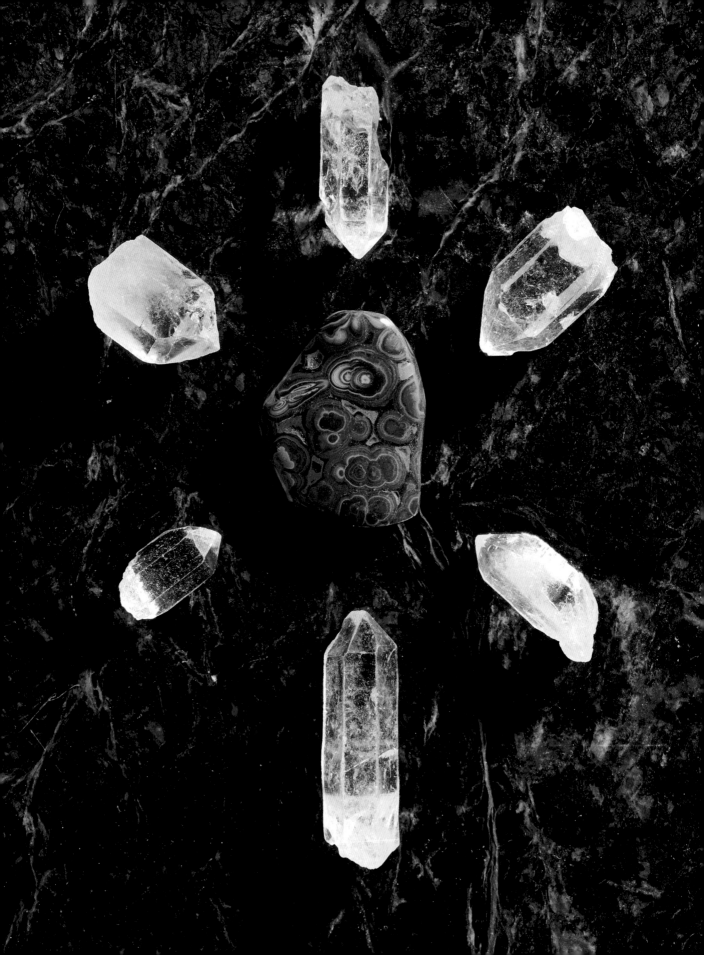

Surround the stone you want to charge
with a minimum of four clear quartz apexes,
points facing the stone.

Once the stone is cleaned, the next step is to charge or program it using your personal energy as well as that of sunlight and other crystals. Start by setting your intention. (In other words, what are you hoping to achieve?) Take the stone in your left hand, placing your right hand over it, and make your intention known by either stating out loud or thinking to yourself your purpose in using the stone.

Next, let the sun do its job and place the stone or stones on a sunny windowsill or in any spot that receives direct sunlight. The sun's rays are very energizing as well as energetically clearing. Leave stones there for a minimum of twenty-four hours, or up to a week. But check on them regularly, since some colors will fade in direct sunlight. Stones such as amethyst, celestite, kunzite, opal, and turquoise may be charged in moonlight. If you have any doubts at all, let the moon do the charging—or place the stone under a full-spectrum lightbulb or plant light for an hour.

Another way to charge or program a stone is by using natural clear quartz apexes, also known as quartz points, to form what's called a quartz circle. Apexes are short crystal rods with one pointed end. Simply surround the stone you want to charge with a minimum of four clear quartz apexes, points facing the stone. Leave the circle in place for at least twenty-four hours. If you don't have access to apexes, you can also use a houseplant. Just place the gemstone at the base of a healthy plant for twenty-four hours or more. You can also charge your crystals with a clear quartz crystal cluster. Additionally, you can try putting the crystals in the ocean and/or sand (try putting them in a piece of cotton or a pouch). A pyramid is another great way to charge crystals; place your crystal(s) in a pyramid for no more than 12 hours.

If you're looking to clear and charge smoky quartz or any dark, opaque crystal or gem, you can bury it just below the surface of a dirt-filled flowerpot (with or without a plant) for a week or more.

A TOOL NAMED FOR TESLA

If you're looking to speed up your charging process, a device called a purple plate comes in tremendously handy. In fact, placing crystals and gemstones on such a plate for twelve hours energizes them in a fraction of the time it usually takes.

What is this magical device? A purple plate is a thin, typically square-shaped aluminum plate ranging in size from a 1-inch to a 12-inch square that has been anodized (a process that uses chemical baths to prepare the surface of aluminum to receive an electrical charge that increases the thickness of the oxide layer and makes it more durable and less likely to corrode). Through this process of restructuring atoms and electrons, the plates are somehow altered to vibrate at a frequency similar to that of the stones themselves. Manufacturers prefer to keep this process confidential, but whatever they do to them, the plates work! Purple plates are known to raise vibratory frequencies of any living thing, from people to plants to animals. Though purple plates are named for Nikola Tesla—an inventor, electrical and mechanical engineer, and physicist known for his contributions to the design of the modern alternating current (AC) electricity supply, radio, the X-ray, and telecommunications—it is Ralph Bergstresser, a man who once worked with Tesla, who is credited for inventing the plates.

Purple plates have many other uses beyond charging stones:

♦ Keep one in a pocket or purse for more energy. (No body contact is necessary.)

♦ Place one in your refrigerator to keep produce fresh longer.

♦ Put one beneath sick house plants, or water sick plants with water that has been placed overnight on a plate.

♦ Slide one beneath your feet and below your torso when relaxing to help move stagnant energy throughout the body. (They're so thin, you'll barely feel them.) We said earlier that it was not that comfortable when I used them for a treatment.

♦ Place one under the glass bowl you use to make your crystal- or gem-enhanced elixir (see "Mixing Elixirs One of Three Ways," page 80) to reduce the charge time by anywhere from thirty minutes to twelve hours.

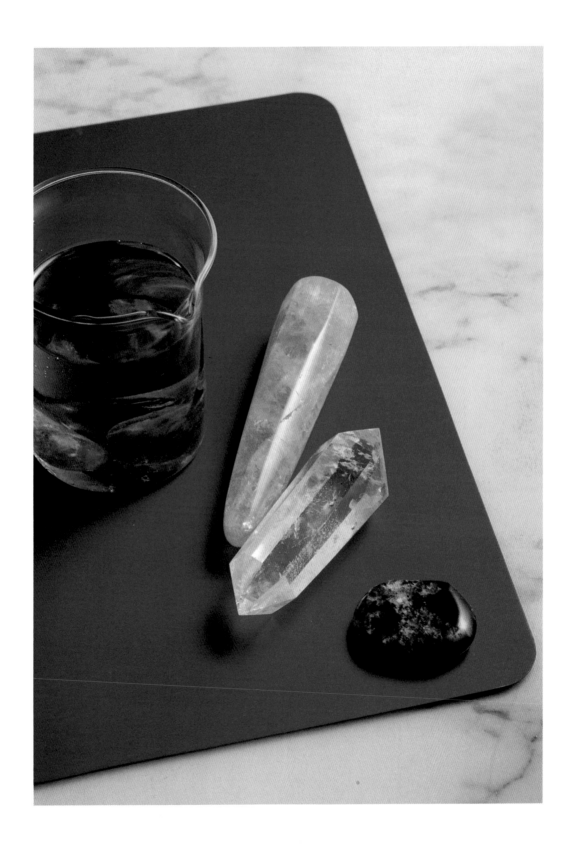

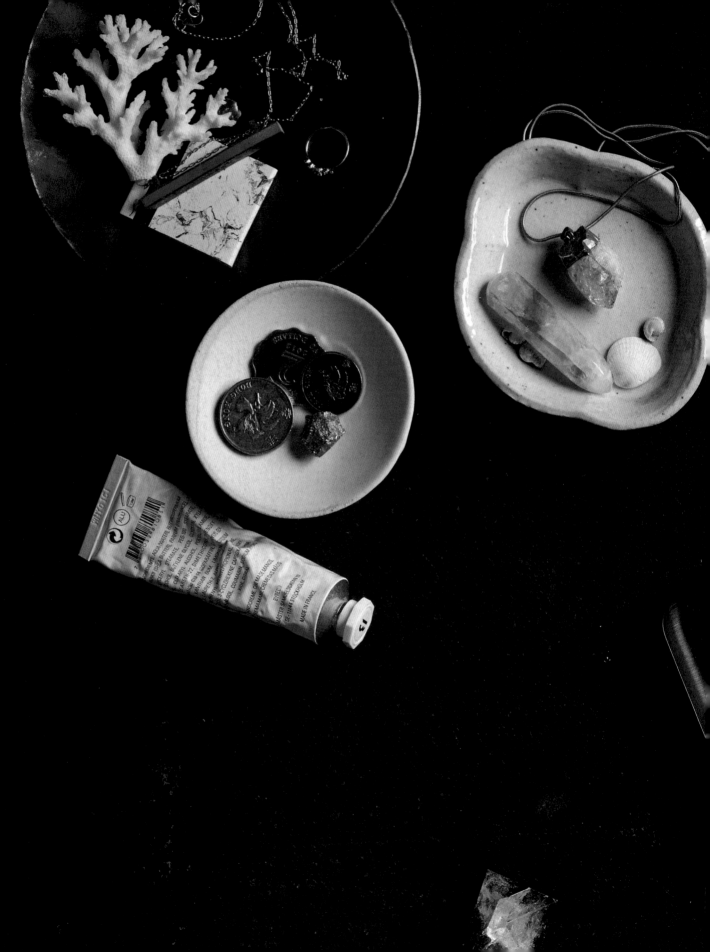

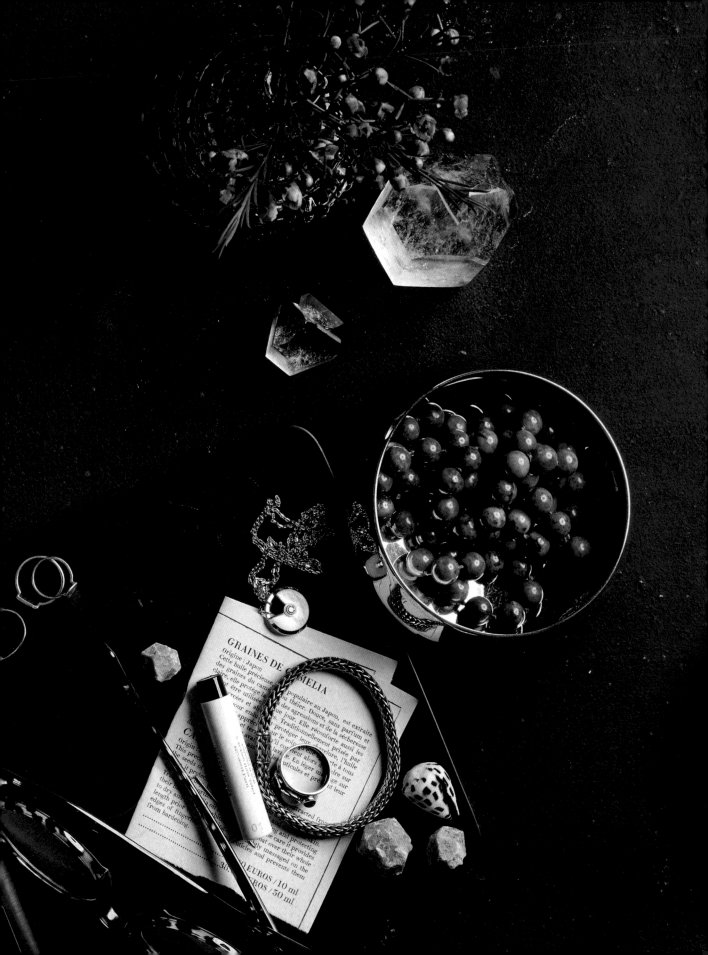

GRAINES DE C...
origine : Japon
Cette huile précieuse ... populaire au Japon, est extraite
des graines du cam... ou théier. Douce, sans parfum et
claire, elle protège la ... des agressions et de la sécheresse
... rcées et a... que jour. Elle réconforte aussi les
... endu... s. Traditionnellement prisée par
... apprecie... protéger leur chevelure, l'huile
... ... er le soin ... ... dre sur
... ... e. En léger m... ... ge sur
... ... ut leur

C... ...
Origin ...
This preci... ...
the seeds of ...
... it protec... ...
... ...
their ... ...
to dry an... ...
length prior ... a oi... ...
edges of fin... ... ...
from hardening. ... ... and protecting.
... ... e care it provides.
... ... lly massaged on the
... ... uticles and prevents them

38. ... EUROS /10 ml
... ROS /50 ml

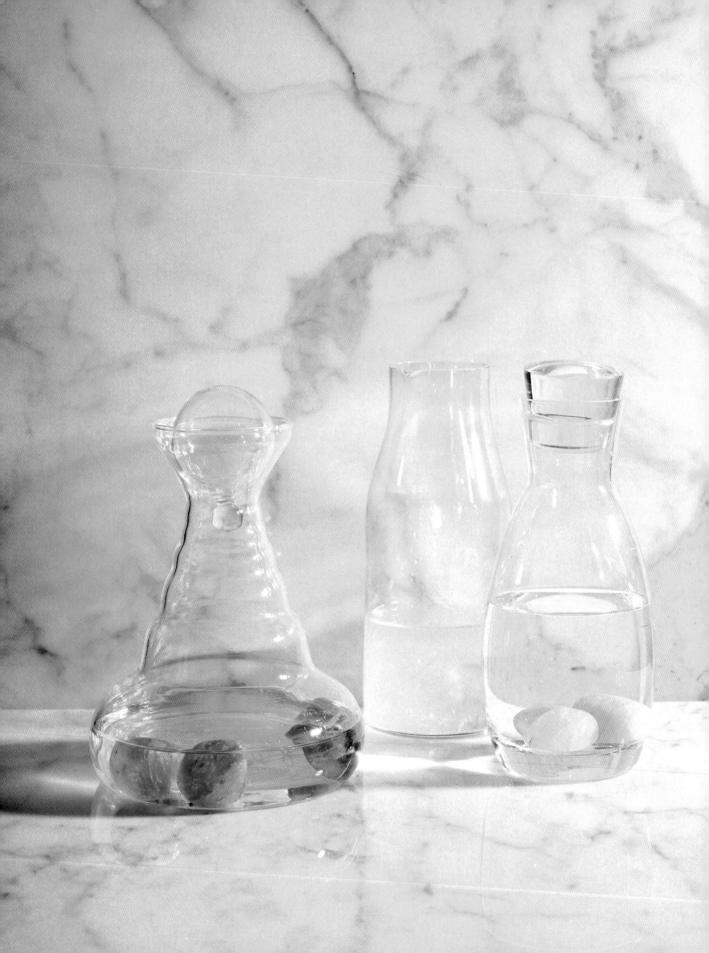

4

ELIXIRS

WATER AND GEMS IN HARMONY

I f you're anything like me, the word "elixir" may at first conjure up the image of a magical potion that grants its drinker eternal life. Of course, no one's been able to come up with that holy grail in a bottle—yet. But as I learned when my mother and I began using gemstone elixirs in our skincare products, though they may not be exactly magical, elixirs *are* an effective, convenient way to infuse lotions, serums, and tonics with crystal and gemstone energy—without including a stone in each jar of our skincare products.

What exactly are gemstone elixirs? In short, they are liquids (typically water or oils) that, through a process you can easily do yourself at home, are imprinted with a particular stone's vibrational energy. When absorbed by the skin during skin treatments, massages, or baths, your body responds to that crystalline energy.

Initially, my mother and I did consider including a physical stone in our products. A crystal and gemstone healer we knew suggested that we incorporate blue sapphire in our skincare. The rationale was that since the stone is known to clear both the mind and the body, perhaps it could also work well on skin. Curious, I did some research and learned that blue sapphire is believed to stimulate the pituitary gland, producing a calm, meditative state. I loved the idea of enhancing our products with the energy of sapphires, since who doesn't look better on the outside when they feel calm and relaxed?

But how would we get the benefits of the stones into the products? At the time, vendors didn't sell crushed gemstone powders, and I decided to turn to the ancients for my answer.

From ancient Egyptians to Benedictine saints, healers routinely soaked crystals and gem-stones (along with herbs and other plant matter) in water or oil and used the sun's heat to charge them. They then relied on these gem-infused liquids to heal, cure, and, in some instances, connect their users to a higher power. Why would that have been effective? Well,

CARRIER OILS 411

What are carrier oils? Carrier oils are vegetable oils derived from the fatty portion of a plant, typically from its seeds, kernels, or nuts. They get their name from their use in aromatherapy, in which carrier oils are used to dilute essential oils prior to topical application. (Applying essential oils directly to the skin can cause severe irritation and is therefore a definite don't!)

How do carrier oils work? When skin absorbs carrier oils charged with crystals or gemstones, the vibrational energy of the elixir is believed to be transferred to the skin on a subtle level.

Which carrier oils should you use? First, you want to look for carrier oils that have been cold-pressed. This means that the oil has been extracted from the botanical without the use of heat (which can damage the integrity of the oil), making it the richest in vitamins, minerals, and proteins. Also, different oils have different levels of viscosity, which determines how they feel on the skin. You may want to use lighter oils on the face for better penetration and absorption, and heavier oils on the body. Here are quick groupings of lighter and heavier oils for use in crafting elixirs:

LIGHTER OILS	HEAVIER OILS
Grape seed	Sweet almond
Evening primrose	Avocado
Apricot kernel	Coconut
Meadowfoam seed	Macadamia nut
Camilla seed	Olive oil
Jojoba	Rosehip seed

You can combine various oils to create blends. Try blending a lighter and heavier oil to start. Once you're more familiar with the various oils, you can mix and match as you please.

You can custom-create a crystal or gemstone concoction that will resonate with you, whether you need an infusion of calming or elevating energy.

when you soak crystals and gemstones in liquid, the sun's heat fosters the transference of the stone's energy to the liquid so that you capture the energetic blueprint, essence, or life force of a stone.

As I mentioned earlier, making gemstone elixirs is pretty simple. It involves soaking stones in liquid (traditionally water) for a period of time, allowing the sun to charge the liquid by imprinting it with the stones' energy, and then removing the stones. There are three ways to get the job done effectively: Submerging the stone directly in liquid is referred to as the direct method; putting some sort of barrier (such as a drinking glass) between the stone and the liquid is called the indirect method. The third, less common, method, involving boiling the stone in water and hence called the boiling method, yields similar results in less time.

Truthfully, I almost always use the direct method, but if you're at all concerned about the toxicity of certain stones, the indirect method adds a layer of safety, as does boiling the elixir. When I make elixirs, I use either water or carrier oils such as grape seed or sweet almond for the liquid base. The carrier oils work well with skin because they're hydrating, nourishing, and easily absorbed. In addition, many of the oils have antibacterial, antifungal, and antiviral properties.

MAKING GEM ELIXIRS AT HOME

Making your own elixirs at home requires more time than energy (yours, not the stone's). But in doing so, you can custom-create a crystal or gemstone concoction that will resonate with you, whether you need an infusion of calming or elevating energy. What's more, you can mix several crystal- or gem-enhanced elixirs simultaneously so you'll have them on hand for all of the massage, skincare, and bath treatments that you'll find in subsequent chapters. Water elixirs also make great room sprays or refreshing spritzes for face and body, so have fun experimenting and observing how your mind and body react in response to the various vibrational frequencies of different stones.

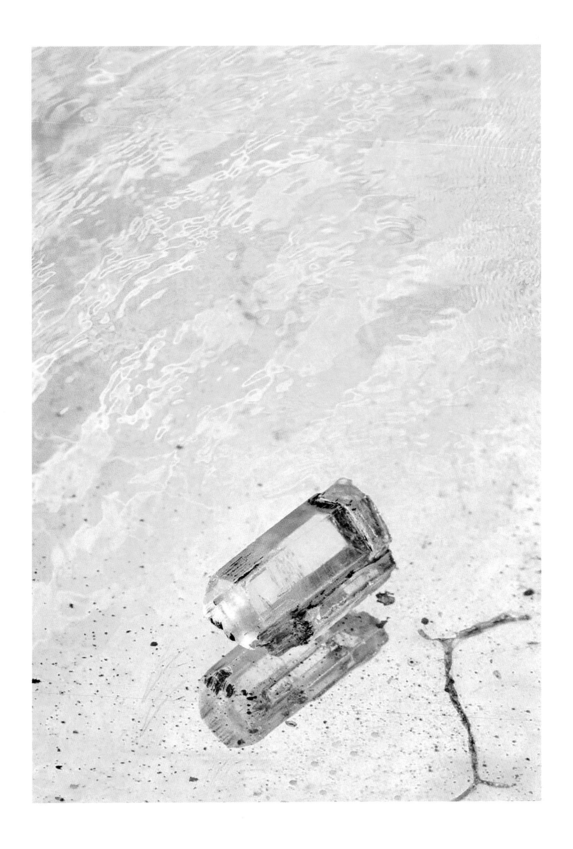

Ready to start mixing a custom elixir? Here are the supplies you'll need for all three methods (direct, indirect, or boiling):

- Large, clear glass bowl

- Crystal or gemstone (tumbled are best, so points or edges won't break off)

- Glass jar, container, or decorative bottle with a lid (see "Clear Choices," page 79)

- Labels for bottles

- Juice or rocks glass (for the indirect method; it should be large enough to hold a crystal or gemstone)

- Pot with a ceramic interior (for the boiling method)

- 8–16 ounces distilled water or 8–16 ounces carrier oil

- Cheesecloth (should be large enough to cover the glass jar or container to help prevent particles from contaminating the elixir while it charges; can also use a jar with a transparent lid, as long as it's not plastic)

- Elastic band (to secure the cheesecloth to the top of the glass jar or container)

- Vegetable glycerin (to help stabilize the water elixir)

- Wooden spoon (for placing and removing the stones and to keep the crystal from absorbing your own energy and affecting the elixir)

- Full-spectrum lightbulb (if charging your elixir in indirect sunlight, the bulb will help enhance the charge)

What exactly is a tumbled stone? Some stones are naturally smoothed and rounded by remaining under fast-flowing streams of water for long periods of time. This effect can be re-created by placing a rock or mineral in a device called a tumbler, which smooths the stone mechanically and enhances its luster.

Most of the bath and tonic recipes in this book require ½ cup or less of elixir, so 16 ounces of elixir will be enough for four treatments (16 fluid ounces = 2 cups). You always want to make sure that your gem water elixirs are as fresh as possible.

All right, you've gathered your supplies. Now, before you begin crafting your elixir, you need to take these four important steps:

1. Cleanse your stone

After you choose the gemstone or crystal that you would like to charge—
I recommend charging just one stone at a time—use the cleaning methods
from chapter 3 to cleanse away any impurities as well as negative energy.

2. Set your intention

Take a moment to center yourself and think purposefully about why you're
mixing the elixir, the qualities of the stone or stones you are using, and how you
hope the elixir will benefit you. Remember, it is always your intentions that guide
your actions, whether or not you're aware of them. You can even write down an
affirmation and tape it to your glass if you so choose.

3. Get in the mood

When mixing elixirs, it's best to be in a calm state of mind and allow yourself to
enjoy the experience. So if you've had a rough day, try this breathing exercise
before you start mixing: Inhale to the count of five, hold your breath for five
counts, and exhale for five counts. Repeat five times.

4. Sterilize your tools

Use rubbing alcohol to wipe down any bowls, jars, and drinking glasses you'll be
using, then allow them to dry.

Next, depending on your intended usage, you'll choose the liquid that will serve as the base for your elixir.

WATER

Charge time: 3 to 12 hours; 7 hours is optimal
Water elixir uses: Facial recipes, baths, and room sprays

The greatest conductor of energy, water is by far the most commonly used element when it comes to elixirs. It absorbs the properties of the gemstone or crystal placed in it quicker than other liquids do. A growing body of scientific research has uncovered some interesting properties of water that help to explain why, when used in elixirs, water is able to effectively absorb the energy from a crystal or gemstone submerged within it.

One explanation is that water is actually responsive to thoughts and emotions. While this may sound far-fetched, a major proponent of this theory, Dr. Masaru Emoto (1943–2012), devoted his life to "listening" to what water had to say.

In the lab, Dr. Emoto exposed distilled water to positive and negative words, messages, photos, and music before freezing it, and then studied the crystals that formed as a result once the water was solid. For example, he would tape a note with the words "thank you" on one bottle of water and later observe delicate, symmetrical crystalline shapes under a microscope, whereas a note with a negative message would result in chaotic, fragmented structures that lacked symmetry. The same held true when he exposed the water to consonant and dissonant music. Again and again, he tested his theory, and the results appear to bear out that, indeed, water responded to the various stimuli. Whether you choose to view Dr. Emoto's images as scientific evidence or simply works of art, his theory may help to explain why the water in elixirs "embraces" the positive energy within a stone and holds it dear before "sharing" it with the user.

CLEAR CHOICES

When it comes to charging and storing your elixirs, you'll want to use a glass jar or other glass container with a lid, but other than that, the sky's the limit. Here are a few suggestions:

Glass carafes: They make for a pretty pour. You can even find one with a "Flower of Life" sacred symbol etched into the base. What better way to amp up the energy in your elixir?

Milk bottles: Just like the milkman used to deliver, these come with stoppers attached.

Apothecary bottles: Dark blue or brown ones are great for storing oil-based elixirs.

Canning or mason jars: Yes, the same jars you use for jams and pickles can be used for elixirs. If you use them to charge your elixir, simply place the cheesecloth under the metal lid.

Glass spray bottles or misters: When filled with a water-based elixir, these can be used to cleanse a room. (Black tourmaline is an ideal stone for this; citrine elixir can be used to clear your mind and improve focus.)

CARRIER OILS

Charge time: A minimum of 12 hours for lighter oils; up to 28 days for heavier ones

Oil elixir uses: Face and body recipes and gemstone facial massages

Natural, organic fatty oils called carrier oils are used as the base for gem elixirs. They are excellent emollients for softening and smoothing skin. Oils take more time to charge than water, as they are composed of larger, denser molecules that take longer to absorb the vibrational energy pattern of gemstones.

MIXING ELIXIRS ONE OF THREE WAYS

Now it's time to mix and charge your elixirs. This is the part when you're combining one or more stones with your chosen liquid, then relying on either the sun or your stove to program the liquid with crystal or gemstone energy.

When making and charging elixirs, you can choose between the direct, indirect, and boiling methods.

For the ***direct method,*** submerge the stones in water or a carrier oil until the liquid is imprinted with the stone's energy.

1. Fill a sterilized glass vessel of your choosing with distilled water.

2. Using a wooden spoon, gently place one cleansed stone in the liquid.

HOLD THE WATER

Certain stones such as, but not limited to, azurite, galena, and cinnabar contain known toxins and should not be used in the direct method. Please check sources before using any stones for gem elixirs—it is always a good idea to check with multiple sources.

Stones such as halite, selenite, lapis lazuli, and turquoise are water-soluble (meaning they're porous and will eventually dissolve in water) and should not be used for elixirs made with the direct method (but they'll work well with the indirect method). Rose quartz, amethyst, and clear quartz are considered safer choices for direct-method elixir making, both in terms of water solubility and toxicity.

3. Secure a piece of cheesecloth over the opening of the vessel with an elastic band.

4. Place the glass vessel outside in the sun (or on a windowsill in direct sunlight), and charge between 3 and 12 hours. If you charge your elixir in indirect sunlight, a full-spectrum lightbulb will help further enhance the charge.

5. Once the elixir is charged, use a clean, sterile wooden spoon to remove the stone, and add 4 to 6 drops vegetable glycerin per 2 cups water to help stabilize the stone's vibration. (You can place the stone in direct sunlight for several hours to reenergize it after adding the glycerin.)

6. Label the elixir, cover, and refrigerate; it can last up to 2 weeks.

7. You can use 4 natural quartz apexes pointing toward the jar in the refrigerator to help it stabilize and charge.

For the **indirect method,** separate the liquid from the stones with a glass barrier. This is considered the safer method. While direct immersion may yield slightly more potent elixirs, indirect immersion provides peace of mind.

1. First, find a drinking glass that will fit inside a glass bowl. It shouldn't be too much taller than the bowl, if it all. Using a wooden spoon, gently place a cleansed stone in the drinking glass, and place the glass in the bowl.

2. Fill the bowl with your chosen liquid to about halfway up the outside of the glass.

3. Use a large piece of cheesecloth and drape it over the glass and the bowl, securing it with a large rubber band.

Next, follow step 4 from the direct method, then remove the drinking glass and stone, and add glycerin to the charged elixir. Transfer the elixir from the bowl to a container with a lid before storing, and follow steps 6 and 7 above.

> To amplify your elixir's energy, surround the glass vessel or bowl with four to twelve clear quartz apexes (aka quartz points), tips facing inward, as the elixir charges.

For the **boiling method,** which is used only for water-based elixirs, bring the liquid—with the stones submerged in it—to a slow and gentle boil. This method is both effective and fast, and doesn't require direct sunlight.

1. Fill a pot with approximately 8 to 16 ounces of distilled water. Using a wooden spoon, gently place one or more cleansed stones in the water.

2. Set the pot over medium to medium-low heat. As soon as the water reaches a slow, gentle boil, remove the pot from the heat source.

3. Let both the water and stones cool to room temperature. Gently pour the water, along with the stones, into a glass vessel.

4. Secure a piece of cheesecloth over the opening of the vessel with an elastic band. If desired, charge the vessel in direct sunlight for at least 4 hours and/or charge with 4 natural crystal points or apexes pointing toward the elixir.

5. Once the elixir is charged, use a clean, sterile wooden spoon to remove the stones, and add 4 to 6 drops vegetable glycerin per 2 cups water to help stabilize the vibration. (You can then place the stones in direct sunlight for several hours to reenergize them after adding the glycerin.)

6. Label the elixir, cover, and refrigerate for up to 2 weeks.

MIXING OIL-BASED ELIXIRS

Although the direct method is typically used to make oil-based elixirs, the process is a bit different from making water-based ones. How so? Well, there are three primary differences:

- Time: Elixirs made with carrier oils take longer to charge than those made with water or aloe. They need to be kept in direct sunlight for a minimum of 12 hours and up to 28 days.

- Preservation: You don't need to add vegetable glycerin to oil-based elixirs to help stabilize them as you do for water-based elixirs.

- Storage: In general, oil-based elixirs do not require refrigeration and have a shelf life of about a year. More delicate carrier oils—such as rosehip seed oil or evening primrose—do require refrigeration and have a shorter shelf life of about six months.

> Once you've created various gemstone and crystal elixirs, experiment with combining them. Try them alone first and take note of how you respond. Then do the same with various combinations until you find your ideal gemstone or crystal "cocktail."

ARE DIY ELIXIRS WORTH THE EFFORT?

In a word, yes. The slow process of charging elixirs may at first be frustrating, given the frenetic pace of daily life in our culture. But just think how long it took for the gems to form! Taking the time to mix your own elixir is a good opportunity to slow down and think about what you're feeling at the moment and which crystals and gemstones might serve to counterbalance those emotions. Plus, it will help you to value the elixir even more once you use it. Although I've been making my own for years, I love seeing how enhancing them with different stones changes the way my skin—and my mind—react.

ESSENTIAL OIL–SCENTED ELIXIRS

Want a wonderful-smelling oil elixir to use daily on your body as a postshower moisturizer? Add a few drops of an essential oil to your oil elixir an hour before taking the stone out—as a rule, use 3 to 6 drops of essential oil per ounce of carrier oil. Never apply undiluted essential oils directly to the skin! For maximum benefit, choose an essential oil that complements the gem in your elixir. Here are some suggestions:

GEM	ESSENTIAL OIL
Rose quartz	Rose, gardenia, tuberose, or ylang-ylang
Moss agate	Pine, eucalyptus, rosemary, or basil balsam
Amethyst	Lavender, frankincense, or myrrh
Citrine	Chamomile or rose
Sapphire	Chamomile or lavender

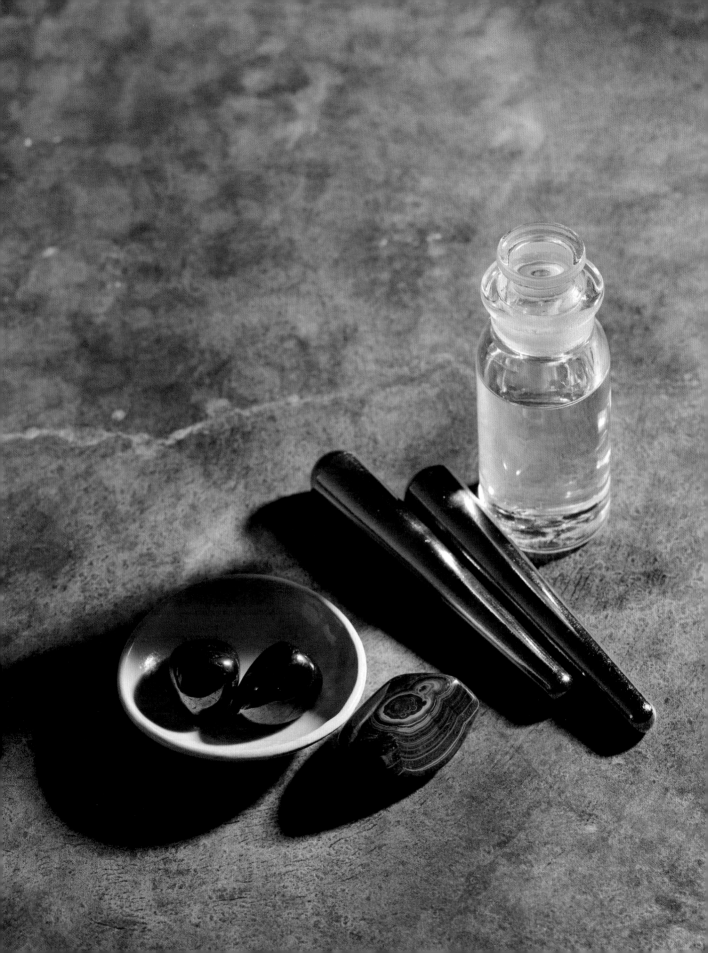

5

IN AN INSTANT

QUICK GEMSTONE AND CRYSTAL MASSAGES

Now that you've learned about some of the properties crystals and gemstones possess and how to infuse water and carrier oils with their energy, it's time to experience the positive, healing powers of crystals and gemstones (along with gem and crystal elixirs) directly. One of the easiest ways I've found to combat stress and balance my emotions is to use specific crystals and gemstones—either tumbled stones or healing wands with one narrow and one broader end—to massage face, hands, and feet using age-old Eastern healing therapies. Gemstone and crystal massages can help you release any physical or emotional tension, or stress, for weeks, months, or even years.

The treatments that follow are rooted in two practices from Traditional Chinese Medicine—acupressure and reflexology—that have been used for thousands (yes, *thousands*) of years to prevent illness and treat chronic conditions. Acupressure is similar to acupuncture, but instead of using needles to stimulate pressure points along the body, therapists apply pressure to those points using their fingers. Here, we'll be using a gemstone or crystal wand. Applying pressure to these points can increase energy and feelings of well-being, while at the same time reducing stress and strengthening the immune system.

Reflexology, a therapeutic technique involving touch therapy that has been traced to predynastic China (possibly as early as 3000 BCE) and to ancient Indian medicine, relieves pain by stimulating specific pressure points on the feet and hands. These points are thought to connect directly through the nervous system to specific organs and glands. Like acupressure, reflexology is considered by many to be effective for promoting good health and preventing illness.

What I find wonderful about the techniques used in the treatments that follow is that they don't require a huge time commitment to be effective. With both acupressure and reflexology, you can see or feel a noticeable difference in just five or ten minutes—further proof that you don't have to invest a lot of time in yourself to achieve results.

Though acupressure and reflexology are usually performed with bare hands, introducing crystals and gemstones to the equation elevates the experience by channeling healing energy to where you need it most. The gemstones and crystals can be used for a multitude of treatments that improve energy flow and leave you feeling relaxed or recharged in a matter of minutes. And if you *are* planning to incorporate at least one of the treatments in this chapter into your self-care regimen, I hope you'll consider purchasing a tumbled stone or crystal wand. Typically, one end of the elongated crystal wand is pointed and the other is rounded, but wands are also available with two rounded ends (one broad, one narrow), which I highly recommend because the sharp points on pointed wands can break off and aren't necessary for the treatments in this chapter.

Why do you need a wand? In addition to helping you apply slightly more pressure than you can with your hands in both acupressure and reflexology treatments, the tool enables the gemstone or crystal to direct its energy to specific areas of the body or

GROUNDING WANDS
Black tourmaline, hematite, and smoky quartz

BALANCING AND CALMING WANDS
Amethyst, rose quartz, sodalite, and scolecite

NEUTRAL WANDS
Moss agate, rose quartz, and moonstone

STIMULATING AND INVIGORATING WANDS
Clear quartz and copper

chakras. And while you may ultimately want to have a collection of wands (which can also sub in for tumbled stones, as needed), you need only one to get started. Clear quartz, rose quartz, or amethyst makes a great starter wand to treat all areas of the body.

Before you use a wand, you should clean and charge it just as you would any stone (see "Bringing Home Your Crystals and Gems," page 64). You'll also want to spend some time familiarizing yourself with its cylindrical shape, texture, and weight. You can hold it while you meditate (see page 200), or just carry it around. Holding the wand will help you become attuned to it, and at the same time you will also receive its healing energies. Don't forget to set an intention for the wand by either speaking out loud or thinking to yourself how you want to use it. (You can always change your intention after cleaning and recharging the wand for future use.)

Which wand you choose for a treatment really depends on what you're trying to accomplish. Certain wands have balancing and calming properties, while others stimulate and invigorate. If you have sensitive skin, I'd advise you to steer clear of more stimulating stones. Otherwise, you can experiment and see which wands provide the desired effect on your face, hands, and feet.

The first time I received a facial massage with a crystal wand was in 2008 when I was working with a hotel group to create a restorative crystal healing facial. Although I was a bit nervous as we were charting unknown territory, I had a great esthetician, Aida, who was ready to help take on this challenge. Aida and her team in Miami had begun working on some massage techniques, and when I arrived at the spa, she had me lie down on the massage table and used a rose quartz wand to perform a very slow circular massage that felt like raindrops on my Third Eye. I had never experienced anything like it. After fifteen minutes I was in a calm, tranquil, almost meditative state. Any signs of stress or anxiety had melted away; I was transformed.

Of course, on that day, and every time I've had an incredible massage or reflexology treatment since, I've sworn that I will make it a regular habit, once a week or at the very least once a month. But even with the best of intentions, life gets in the way. I get it—finding time for self-care is difficult. But in the end, I've come to realize that it's worthwhile for me to carve out ten to fifteen minutes every day to unplug and recharge my emotional battery—and that I don't have to seek professional help to do it. When I make the time for self-care, I have more energy and focus overall, and that makes me a better wife, parent, daughter, and business partner. I'd love it if we all could take that time to check in with ourselves every day: to pause, listen to ourselves, and take just a few minutes to treat ourselves to a simple but truly restorative massage—and I hope that the massages that follow empower you to do just that.

STONES TO TRY

Using various gemstone or crystal wands or tumbled stones will allow you to customize your treatment for a truly healing experience. Here are just a few suggestions, but feel free to use other stones you have on hand.

If you're feeling . . .	Try . . .
under the weather	amethyst
congested	sodalite
low energy	hematite
you're spending too much time on your laptop and electronic gadgets	malachite
in need of inner peace	rose quartz
in need of a calming and restful night's sleep	scolecite

CHECK IN WITH YOURSELF

So how do you know which of the treatments in this chapter is the right one for you *right now*? Find a quiet place and close your eyes. First ask how you are feeling: Are you blissful, centered, and focused? If not, could you use some grounding, or perhaps a little elevating? Think about how your emotions may be affecting you physically: Are you having trouble sleeping? Are you lethargic or jittery? Has your routine been interrupted by travel, a looming deadline, or family stresses? Do you feel bloated, swollen, or congested? If you're simply feeling off your game, try the treatments in this chapter, which are designed to help balance your energy and reestablish your sense of inner peace.

It may take a few tries to perfect moving the stone or wand gently over the appropriate pressure points, but don't give up. Once you master the movements, you can do them

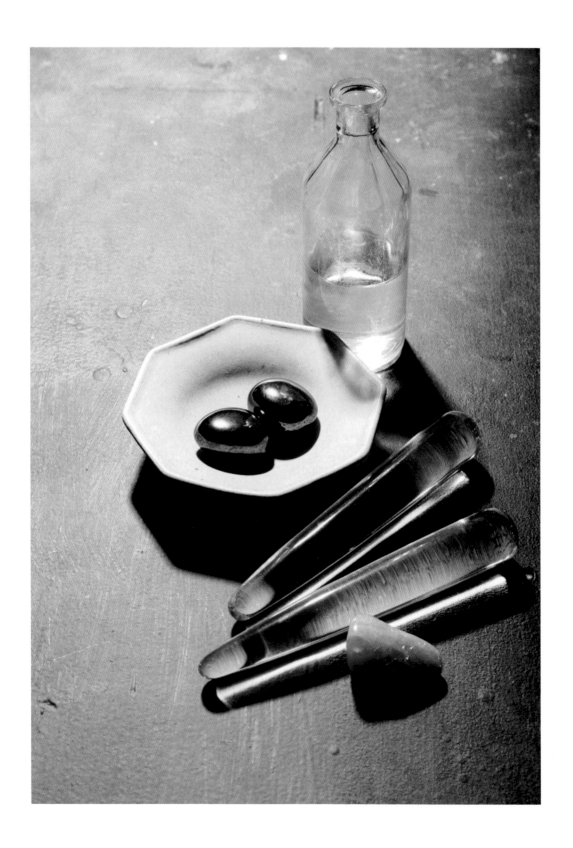

just about anywhere—at home, in an empty office or conference room, or while traveling. You may want to start out doing one or two of these quick and easy treatments a week and work up to more. Feel free to take creative liberties by experimenting with various types of gemstones and crystals (see "Stones to Try," page 88, for ideas). You can also use different oil elixirs in place of the ones I suggest, and face cream will work in a pinch if you haven't mixed any elixirs. In other words, nothing is written in stone. The only thing that is absolute is that the treatments have a calming, healing effect that will make you want to try them again and again. After each treatment, remember to cleanse your crystal, gem, or wand in a nonmetal bowl with warm water and sea salt or on a bed of dry salt for between one and twenty-four hours.

CRYSTAL AND GEMSTONE MASSAGES FOR THE FACE

GEMSTONE WAND FACIAL MASSAGE

If your skin looks as bedraggled as you feel, using a crystal or gemstone wand for this treatment works like magic to bring you and your skin back to life. Whether you're gearing up for an important meeting at work or a big night out, this gentle wand massage increases blood flow, restoring the glow that your skin's been missing. Up the energy ante by customizing the treatment with different stone energies and essential oil–infused elixirs, depending on your state of mind (for ideas, see "Essential Oil–Scented Elixirs," page 83). Once you get the hang of massaging with wands, feel free to get creative, adding your own calming, soothing, and lifting techniques. For example, try using either the broad end or the entire length of the wand to gently release pressure points on your neck and shoulders.

What you'll need:

- 1 or 2 cleansed gem wands, or 1 or 2 tumbled stones, of your choice (see "Stones to Try," page 88). *Note:* For simplicity, the instructions are for two wands. If you use one wand or stone only, repeat each step for each side of the face.

♦ Gem oil elixir to provide slip. The wands should glide, not pull, on skin. If you need more of a glide or a "slip" at any point during your treatment, add a few extra drops of oil.

TIP: For a lighter or more refreshing treatment, or for oily or combination skin, you may want to add a gem water elixir or a tonic; see chapter 8. In a pinch, you can use a facial moisturizer.

Instructions:

1. Follow the diagram on page 92. Apply a few drops of a charged gem oil elixir to cleansed skin. Gently massage the oil elixir into your skin, making sure you evenly distribute the oil to create a slip for the gem wand massage. Towel off your hands and pick up a pair of wands.

2. Hold one wand in your dominant hand. Gently place the broader end of the wand on the Third Eye chakra (at the midpoint of the eyebrows). Make gentle, small circles (the size of a dime) five times clockwise, which helps to bring energy into your body. Keep your focus on the Third Eye. Your forehead is a bone, so go easy and keep the pressure of the wand extremely light. (This massage should feel meditative and tranquil.)

3. Gently place the broad ends of the two wands at the midpoint of the forehead just above the eyebrows (try to keep the wands from touching each other). With light pressure, slowly glide both wands outward toward the temples. Perform your strokes in a gentle, simultaneous, and parallel motion. Return the wands to the starting point. Release the pressure when returning to the start point of each stroke. Repeat three times before progressing up the forehead until you reach the hairline. (Again, this massage should feel meditative and tranquil.)

4. Gently place the broad ends of the two wands under the eyes at the inner corner of the eye area, just under the tear duct. With

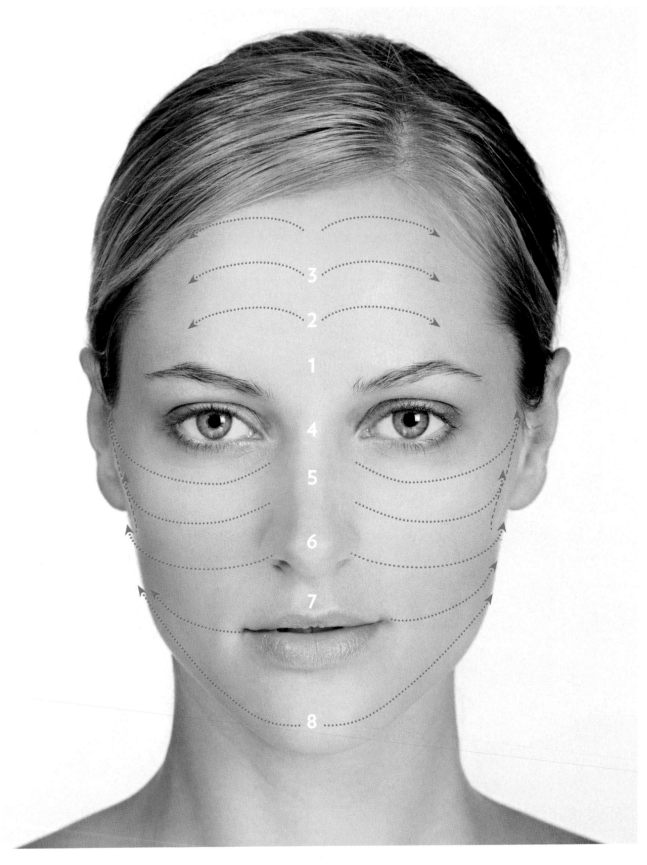

light pressure, using the broad ends, slowly glide both wands outward toward the temples, following the contour of the eyes.

5. Next, place a wand on either side of the bridge of the nose, then glide the broad end of the wand across the cheeks toward the midpoint of the ears in a gentle lifting motion.

6. Gently place a wand on either side of the nostrils. With light pressure, slowly glide both wands outward toward the lobe of the ear, following the contours under the cheekbones. Once you reach the ears, glide the wands down the sides of the face to the point just under the earlobes and behind the jaw, then gently hold and release.

7. Gently place the wands at both corners of the lips. With light pressure, slowly glide the wands to the point under the earlobes and behind the jaw.

8. Gently place the wands at the midpoint of the chin (do not let the wands touch). With light pressure, slowly glide both wands outward to the point under the earlobes and behind the jaw again.

9. Repeat steps 4 through 8 three times.

10. Holding one wand horizontally in the right hand, slowly glide the wand from the side of your right nostril up to the right hairline. Then, using the second wand in the left hand, repeat the upward glide in a slow and consistent manner on the left side of your face. Repeat three times, alternating between the right and left hand.

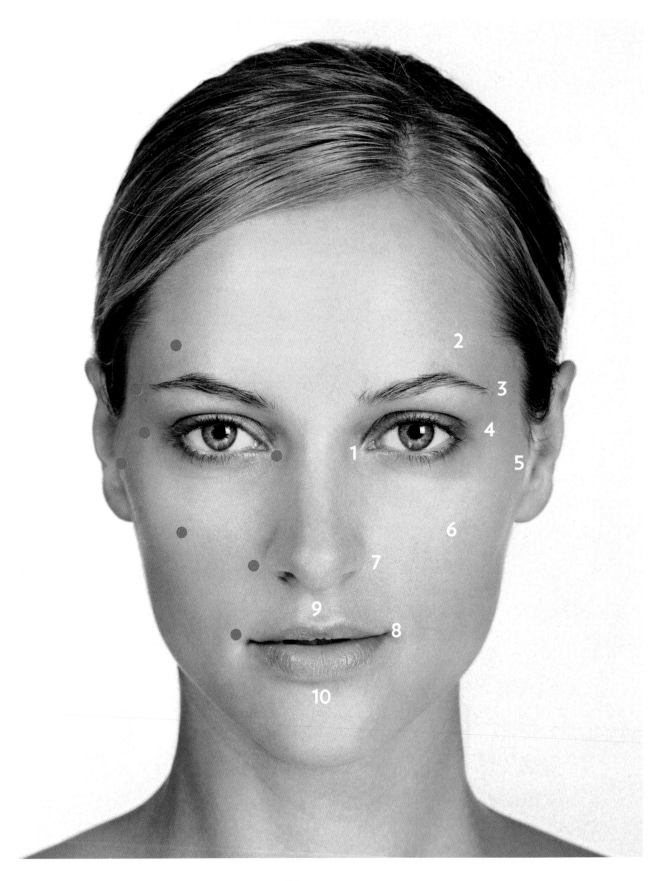

ON-THE-GO ACUPRESSURE FACIAL MASSAGE

The beauty of this ten-minute treatment is that you can do it anywhere. Carry a gemstone wand or stone in your purse and make this your go-to massage during lunch hour, mid-flight, or whenever you need a little pick-me-up. You can customize the treatment by using your favorite stones (see "Stones to Try," page 88).

What you'll need:

♦ Cleansed gem wand or tumbled stone of choice

♦ Gem oil elixir to provide slip, or glide

TIP: For a lighter or more refreshing treatment, or for oily or combination skin, you may prefer to use a gem water elixir or a tonic; see chapter 8. In a pinch, you can use a facial moisturizer.

Instructions:

1. Apply a few drops of a gem oil elixir to cleansed skin. Gently massage the elixir into your skin, making sure you evenly distribute the oil to create slip for the wand or stone.

2. Using either the broad end of a cleansed wand or the smooth side of a cleansed tumbled stone, start on the right side of your face. Follow the point-by-point chart on the facing page using comfortable medium pressure (lighten the pressure in the delicate under-eye area—it should never hurt). Hold each point for approximately 7 to 10 seconds, taking deep breaths as you hold the points. Repeat on the left side of your face.

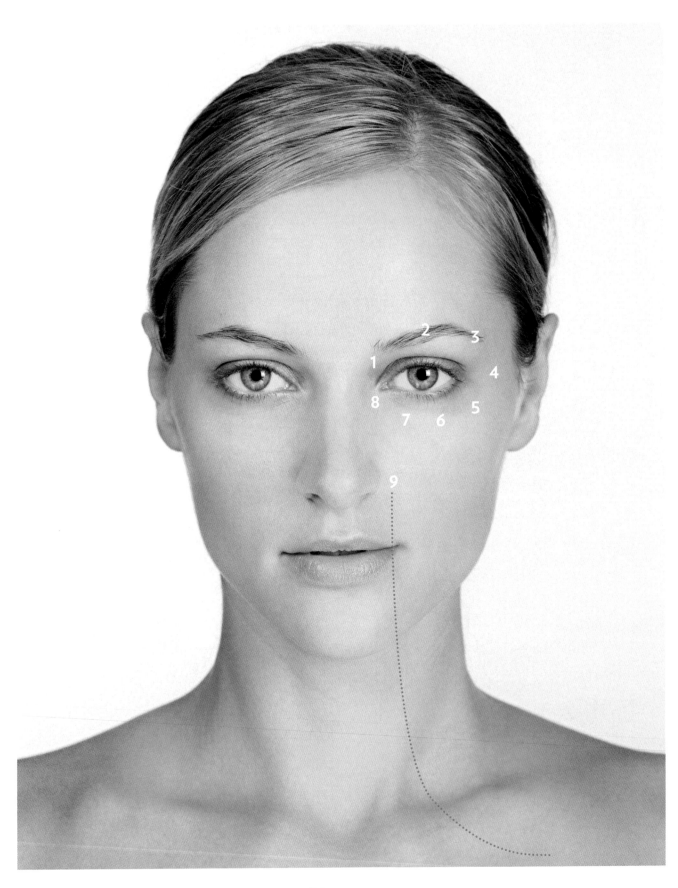

SHIATSU EYE TREATMENT WITH HEMATITE STONES

Late night? I use this morning-after skin treatment to help awaken the area around my eyes by combating puffiness and helping to alleviate dark under-eye circles. (By the way, it's also great for sinus congestion.) Hematite, which is naturally cool to the touch, is 70 percent iron, so it helps blood circulation and is naturally energizing.

What you'll need:

+ Eye cream or charged gem oil elixir
+ 2 tumbled hematite stones

   TIP: Blending a few droplets of oil elixir with your eye cream will help to create a better slip.

Instructions:

1. Gently apply a basic eye cream, gem oil elixir, or a combination of the two to the entire eye orbital area with your ring finger.

2. Take one hematite stone in each hand and, with the rounded edges, press on point 1 as shown on the facing page, applying light to medium pressure. Repeat on points 2 through 8.

3. Move stones down to point 9. Press gently three times.

4. Glide the stones simultaneously from point 9 down the neck to point 10 (a lymphatic point). Press gently and flick to release.

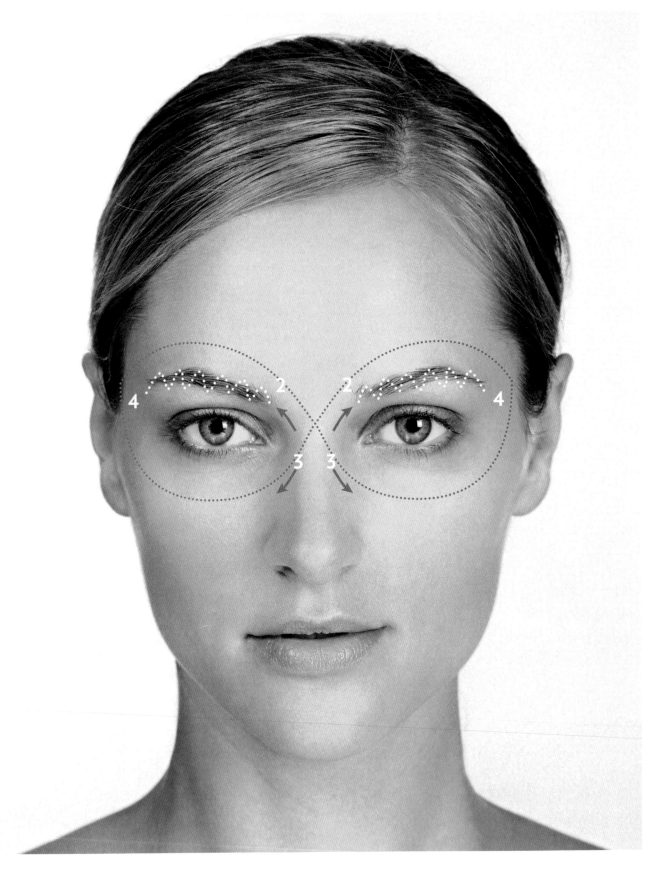

RELAXING DETOX EYE MASSAGE WITH HEMATITE

When you're stressed, it shows in your face, particularly in the sensitive area around the eyes. This treatment helps to combat both emotional and environmental stressors by breaking up any fluid or tension around the eye while also leaving you energized.

What you'll need:

♦ Eye cream or charged gem oil elixir

♦ 2 tumbled hematite stones

Instructions:

1. Gently apply an eye cream, gem oil elixir, or a combination to the entire eye orbital area with your ring finger.

2. Holding a hematite stone in each hand, gently place both stones on the inner edge of the right brow, as marked on the facing page. Applying light pressure, simultaneously move the stones up and down to create a gentle zigzag motion until you reach the outer edge of the brow, making sure the movements are tight and close to each other, hitting on the brow and just slightly above it. Repeat three times on the right side before switching to the left brow.

3. Holding a hematite stone in each hand, place a stone just below each eye orbital and gently move them away from each other and up around the brows, creating an infinity sign (or figure 8) around the eye orbitals.

4. End by gently holding a hematite stone on each temple and applying light pressure. Take a deep breath and hold the stones in place for 5 to 10 seconds. Remove.

ACUPRESSURE FOR WHAT AILS YOU

Once you see how transformative gemstone and crystal massage can be for both your skin and your state of mind, you may want to delve deeper into its therapeutic benefits. Here are three quick facial treatments that use acupressure techniques to help mitigate the symptoms of common ailments, from headaches to anxiety to swelling. Simply use the flat or smooth side of a tumbled gemstone or the broad side of a gemstone wand of choice and gently apply mild to medium pressure, depending on your level of comfort, on the acupressure points described below. Hold the stones on each point for 5 to 10 seconds. Each treatment should be done a minimum of three times in one sitting, but the more the better.

FOR HEADACHE OR INSOMNIA

♦ **Point 1:** M-HN-3 Yin Tang (Hall of Impression), located at the middle of the brow between the eyes (the Third Eye)

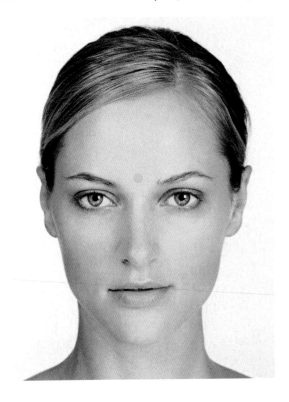

FOR STRESS OR ANXIETY

♦ **Point 1:** Du-24 Shen Ting (Courtyard of the Spirit), located on the midline of the forehead; from the Third Eye (between the eyebrows), go straight up—the point is just at the hairline

♦ **Point 2:** GB-14 Yang Bai (Yang White), located bilaterally on the forehead, directly above the pupil of the eye—one inch or *cun* (Chinese "body inch," which is the width of a thumb) just above the middle of the eyebrow

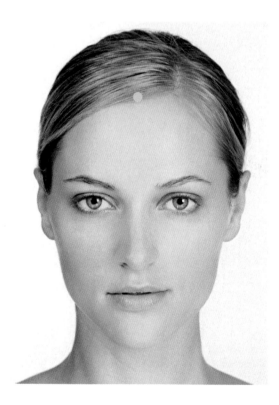
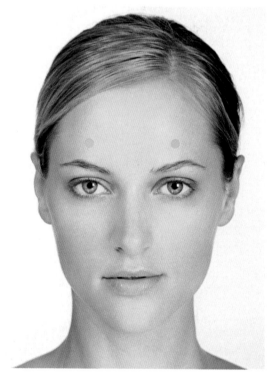

FOR SWELLING

♦ **Point 1:** SI-18 Quan Liao (Cheekbone Crevice), located at the intersection of a vertical line from the outer corner of the eye and the lower border of the cheekbone on the front edge of the jaw muscle (in a slight depression of the lower cheekbone); applying pressure relieves swelling around the eyes and face

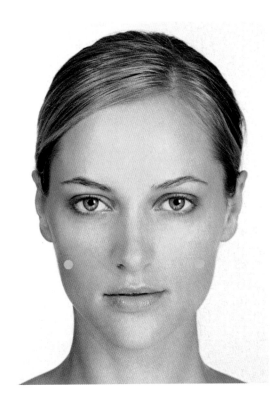

CRYSTAL AND GEMSTONE MASSAGE FOR HANDS AND FEET

These reflexology-inspired treatments for both hands and feet can be used to improve your energy flow and, in turn, your health, by gently manipulating areas of the hand and foot that correspond to organs in the body.

In traditional reflexology treatments, when an organ is not functioning properly, the parts of the foot that correspond to it are sensitive to pressure. Organs that come in pairs (lungs, kidneys, adrenals, and some reproductive organs) are represented on both feet. Other organs, while also represented on both feet, are more strongly reflected on the side on which they are located. The heart, for example, is reflected more strongly on the left foot, and the liver more on the right foot.

Just as the points on both feet correspond to various organs, so do the points on your hands. Once I began to understand these concepts, it was easy to see why reflexology is so much more than just a massage technique.

RELAXING CRYSTAL HAND MASSAGE

By using a stone or wand to stimulate organs—from the pituitary gland to digestive organs to the reproductive system—that correspond with various points in the hands, you have the ability to calm your entire body. Applying medium pressure to these points helps provide a release and relieves tension.

What you'll need:

- Terry cloth towel
- Tumbled stone or gemstone wand
- Gem oil elixir

Instructions:

1. Apply the gem oil elixir to your hands and massage it in to stimulate your circulation. Clean your fingertips on a towel to remove any excess oil; this way you'll be able to get a good grip on the wand or stone.

2. Use the wand or stone to stimulate each of the three zones on the palms of your hands, as per the illustration on the facing page.

3. Slowly glide the wand or stone over each of the zones to warm and condition the muscles. Use small circles to gently knead the muscles, gradually increasing pressure to your comfort level. Lighten pressure over your bones; move slowly and more deliberately over areas that are sensitive.

4. Hold the wand or stone in your dominant hand. Referencing the illustration on the facing page, perform a pressure-point massage to the palm of your left hand. Sink the tip of the wand into the point until you feel a comfortable level of resistance. Hold the point for 7 to 10 seconds, then gently pulse the pressure by alternately holding and releasing the point several times. Slowly release pressure until the wand is no longer in contact with the skin.

5. Repeat on the right hand.

ZONES: HANDS

In reflexology, each area, or zone, of the hand corresponds with different body organs and systems, as follows:

Zone 1: This zone encompasses the lungs, breasts/chest, back, heart (on left palm), shoulders, and arms. Eyes and ears are along the base of the fingers (proximal) where the fingers join to the hands. The tips of the fingers (distal) are the head, brain, and sinus. The neck is located on the fingers between the base and tips.

Zone 2: The right palm encompasses the liver, gall bladder, adrenal glands, colon, kidney, and lymph drainage. The left palm encompasses the stomach, pancreas, spleen, colon, kidney, and lymph drainage.

Zone 3: This zone encompasses the small intestine, bladder, lower back, and spine (on lower right and left palm of hand).

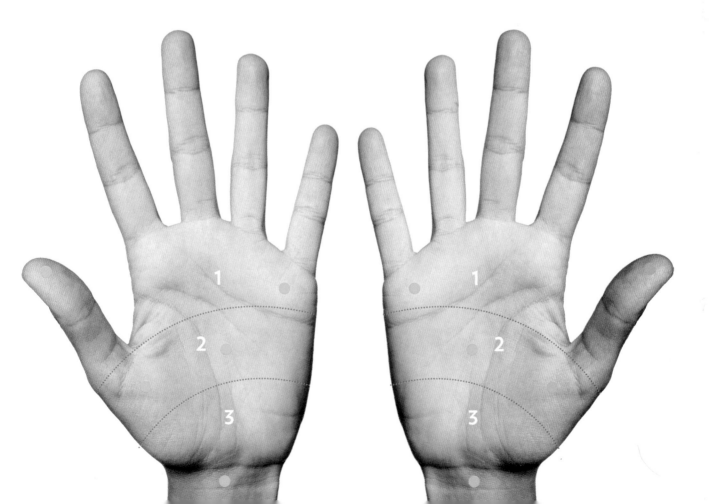

GEMSTONE ENERGY FOOT MASSAGE

This treatment is ideal for tired and achy feet. It helps to break up stagnant energy and alleviate swelling while providing a soothing massage.

What you'll need:

- Grounding gemstone wand
- Gem oil elixir

Instructions:

1. Apply the gem oil elixir to your feet and massage it in to stimulate circulation. Clean your fingertips on a towel to remove any excess oil; this way you'll be able to get a good grip on the wand or stone.

2. Use the wand or stone to stimulate each of the three zones on the soles of your left foot, as per the illustration. Slowly glide the wand or stone over each of the zones to warm and condition the muscles. Use small circles to gently knead the muscles, gradually increasing pressure to your comfort level. Lighten pressure over your bones; move slowly and more deliberately over areas that are sensitive.

3. Next, hold the left foot securely at the base of the heel. With a wand in the other hand, follow the illustration on the facing page to perform a pressure-point massage on the entire sole of the left foot. Sink the tip of the wand into the point until you feel a comfortable level of resistance. Hold the point for 7 to 10 seconds, then gently pulse the pressure by alternately holding and releasing the point several times. Slowly release pressure until the wand is no longer in contact with the skin.

4. Repeat on the right foot.

ZONES: FEET

Zone 1: This zone encompasses the lungs, heart (on the left sole), shoulders, and arms. Eyes and ears are along the base of the toes (proximal) where the toes join to the feet. The tips of the toes (distal) are the head, brain, and sinus. The neck is located on the toes between the base and tips.

Zone 2: The right sole encompasses the liver, gall bladder, adrenal glands, kidney, and pancreas. The left sole encompasses the stomach, pancreas, spleen, adrenal glands, and kidney.

Zone 3: The right sole encompasses the ascending colon, first half of the transverse colon, small intestine, bladder, lower back, hip, knee, ankle, and foot. The left sole encompasses the transverse colon, descending colon, small intestine, bladder, lower back, hip, knee, ankle, and foot.

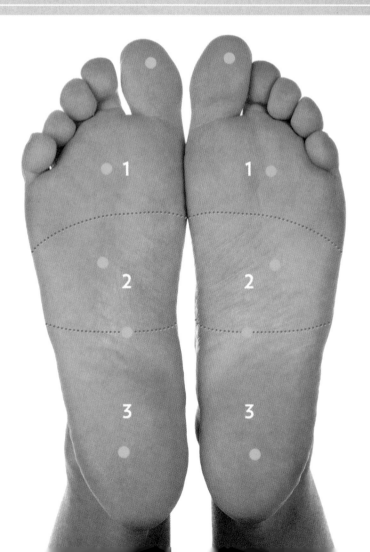

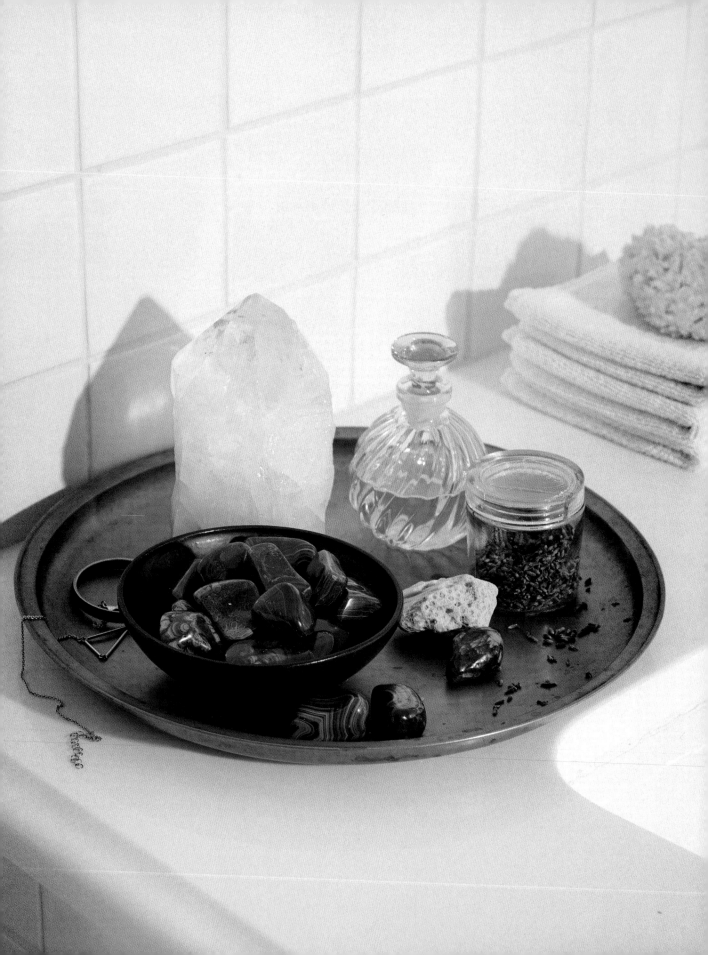

6

BATHING

GEMSTONE THERAPIES AND RITUALS

If you've ever settled into a bath at the beginning or end of a long day, you know how beneficial it can be for putting both your mind and your muscles at ease. The rituals that go hand in hand with bathing—oils, candles, and maybe some relaxing music—all contribute to the overall experience. But the benefits of baths go far beyond their ability to cleanse and calm you. In fact, bathing was widely used in ancient cultures as a therapeutic treatment for body, mind, and spirit.

Ancient Egyptian royalty, who were among the first to identify and understand the beautifying properties of a good bath, bathed with essential oils and flowers (Cleopatra is said to have favored skin-softening milk baths). Some believe that hydrotherapy, a term that refers to the medicinal use of water, got its start even earlier in Asia, where natural hot springs rich in minerals were often used to cleanse the body of impurities.

The ancient Greeks were big believers in the healing power of hydrotherapy. Hippocrates, the physician known as the father of Western medicine, prescribed bathing in spring water for sickness. The Romans borrowed from the Greeks and one-upped them by building large communal bathhouses around hot springs, which were meant as much for socializing as for healing numerous ailments.

The age-old tradition of hydrotherapy continues today. A growing body of research suggests that water therapies (both warm and cool treatments) increase blood circulation, including circulation of the immune system's white blood cells. Bathing in hot water

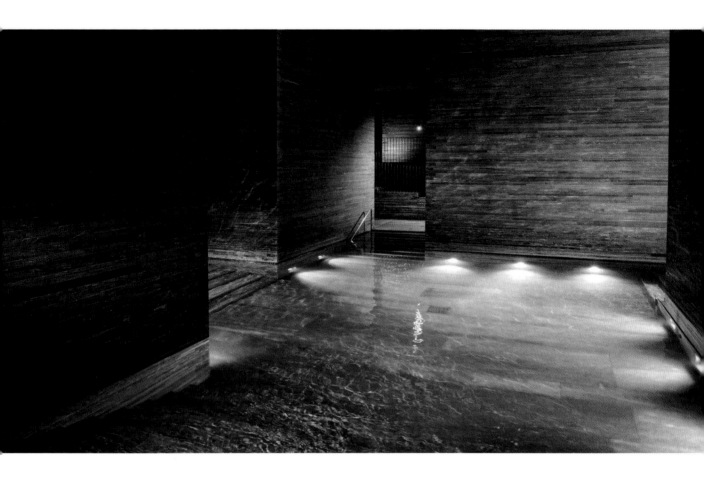

is known to cause organs of the endocrine system to become less active, particularly the adrenal glands, and can decrease blood pressure. Research suggests that water baths also decrease stress hormones like cortisol and balance the feel-good neurotransmitter serotonin. Having trouble getting to sleep? Hot baths are a great alternative to sleeping pills, since the heat temporarily raises body temperature. When you step out of the tub, the drop in your body temperature cues your body to feel sleepy. If you're coming down with a cold, a hot bath can be useful because inhaling hot water vapor (aka steam) causes the small airways and air sacs in the lungs to dilate, increasing the lung's ability to move out phlegm and mucus.

Of course, the reasons for settling into a tub transcend health benefits. Submerging yourself in water also impacts the spirit, as those who flock to natural baths around the world—from Pamukkale hot springs in Turkey to Iceland's Blue Lagoon to the Therme Vals in Switzerland—to experience their healing and purifying properties can attest.

Despite their ability to cleanse the body *and* the soul, baths have been "in" and "out" over the years. After the fall of Rome and during the Middle Ages, the practice of hydrotherapy seemed to disappear. During the medieval era, the Church frowned upon the immorality of bathhouses, and Western doctors actually discouraged taking baths. Fortunately, hydrotherapy was "rediscovered" and popularized in Europe during the Victorian era. By the mid-nineteenth century, the cleanliness of the individual became associated with his or her moral and social standing within the community. During the first half of the twentieth century, some institutions began installing communal baths to help treat children suffering from tuberculosis and polio. It wasn't until the second half of that century, however, that spas began to offer water-based treatments for both healing *and* relaxation.

GEMSTONES, MEET HOT WATER

While mineral baths, such as those offered at many spas, have a long curative history, baths that incorporate crystals and gemstones as part of hydrotherapy treatments are far less common. However, doing so is known to help calm, restore, and detoxify the body on a cellular level. The baths that follow incorporate the healing power of gemstones—good for detoxing, calming, and energizing—in several forms: actual stones, organic gem powders (such as crushed pearl), and gem elixirs. When you try the bath recipes, pay close attention to how you feel so that you can modify them to achieve optimal results. Remember: everyone responds differently to certain stones, so finding the ones that resonate with you, and with which you resonate, requires some trial and error.

Before and as you dive in to these bath treatments, keep in mind a few things:

- To prevent your stones from cracking, begin by running lukewarm, not hot, water. Gently place the stones on the bottom of the tub. Once the stones are fully submerged in water, gradually increase the temperature to moderately hot.

- When adding stones to a bath, caution is necessary, since not all stones do well in hot water for long periods of time. Avoid toxic or soft stones like galena, selenite, malachite, turquoise, and amber. These are best placed around the tub rather than in it.

- As with all of the treatments in this book, finding the ideal stone, combination of stones, or elixir-stone combination for each bath requires a little trial and error. Start by using just one stone or elixir, and each time you try a bath, add another until you find your ideal combination.

- If you prefer to keep your stones in one place while you bathe, place them in a cotton drawstring pouch beforehand. (If you have very small stones, use a tea infuser.)

- Alternatively, if you have loose stones in the bath, feel free to place them on any areas of the body that may feel right for you (e.g., your lower back, stomach, heart, and Third Eye).

- If you're using stones in any bath, always dry them with a soft cloth afterward and place them in a bowl of sea salt overnight to cleanse them.

- You may want to consider using a mesh or silicone drain protector to prevent debris or stones from going down the drain.

- After bathing, *do* lie down for a few minutes with your feet slightly raised (prop a pillow underneath your shins or ankles) to restore proper circulation. *Don't* take a shower. Letting the substance settle into the skin increases the cleansing effect (with the exception of the Detoxifier bath, page 115).

- Feel free to adapt any of these recipes to suit your needs.

- Finally, *bathe sparingly.* A bath takes up to 70 gallons of water, whereas the average shower uses 10 to 25. One or two baths a week will do you good, but do limit the number of baths you take, particularly if you live in a drought-prone area.

- As a precaution, always consult with your doctor if you are on medication, have a chronic condition, or have any concerns before trying the bath recipes in this chapter. Also, it is not advised to take these baths when pregnant.

NO WATER, PLEASE

These stones are porous or water-soluble and you should avoid placing them in your bath:

amber	lapis lazuli	selenite
halite	malachite	turquoise

DRY BRUSHING

As much as we rely on our skin to aid in detoxification and blood flow, we rarely give it the time and attention it deserves. An easy way to do so is to use a technique called dry brushing before getting into the bath (or shower, on days you're not bathing). It's a great prebath ritual for many reasons. For starters, it helps shed dead skin cells while encouraging new cell renewal, which results in smoother and brighter skin. Moreover, dry brushing helps improve vascular blood circulation and lymphatic drainage. By releasing toxins, it encourages the discharge of metabolic wastes so the body is able to run more effectively. And that's not all! Dry brushing rejuvenates the nervous system by stimulating nerve endings and helps skin absorb nutrients by eliminating clogged pores. Ready to get started? Here's how:

What you'll need: A natural-bristle brush (not one made from nylon or synthetic materials) with a long handle, so you can reach all areas of the body

What to do: Brush dry skin before bathing. Work in gentle, circular, upward motions at first, then in longer, smoother strokes. Always begin at the ankles and move up the lower legs, thighs, stomach, and chest toward the heart, because the lymphatic fluid flows in that direction.

One exception: When brushing your back, move in the opposite direction (from the neck down to the lower back). Never brush inflamed skin, sores, sunburned skin, or areas with skin cancer.

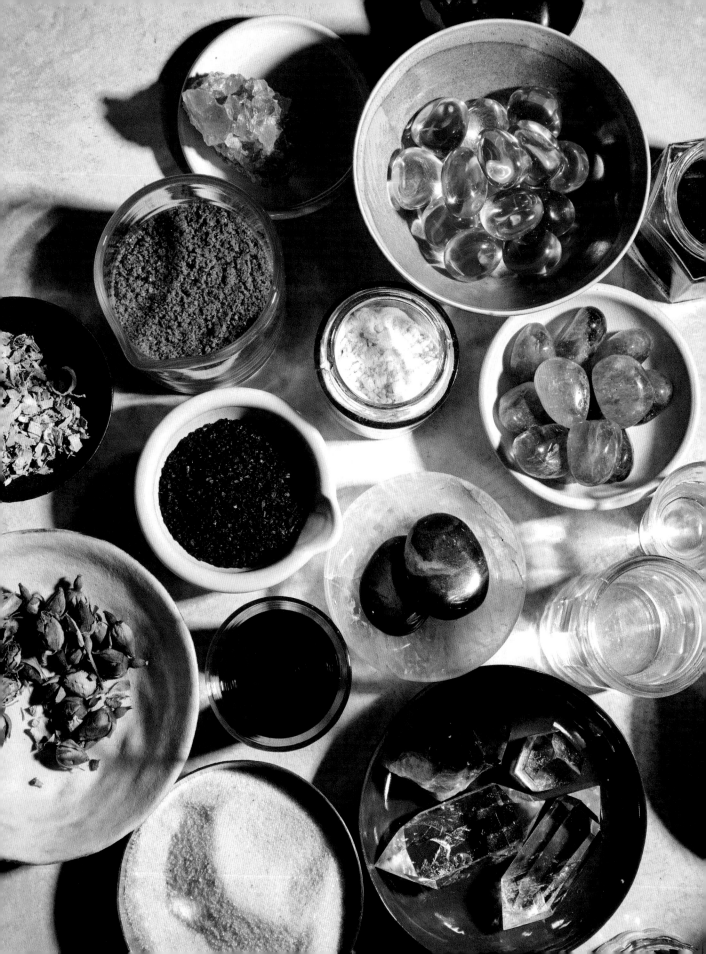

BATH RECIPES

THE DETOXIFIER

This bath works like a magnet to help pull toxins out of the body—the negative charge of the bentonite clay actually bonds with the positive ions in toxins. And the restorative minerals found in clay and sea salt, as well as the alkalizing effects of baking soda, help purify the body. Using black sea salt, which is optional, has an added benefit: the activated charcoal from which it's made assists in releasing impurities. This bath stimulates the lymphatic system and is great for anyone who feels toxic or sluggish or is regularly exposed to heavy metals or EMFs from cell phones, iPads, computers, microwaves, televisions, X-rays, and so forth. You may feel tired after this bath, so do it in the evening before bed no more than once a week. Drink at least one glass of cold water during and immediately after the bath to stay hydrated.

What you'll need:

♦ Suggested stone(s) and/or ½ cup gem elixir: clear quartz, green moss agate, and/or amethyst

♦ 1 cup bentonite clay

♦ ½ cup sea salt or Hawaiian black sea salt

♦ ¼ cup baking soda

Power Ingredient: Bentonite Clay

Composed of aged volcanic ash, bentonite has been used as a detoxifier for centuries. It's powerful stuff: after the meltdown at Chernobyl, Russian crews used bentonite clay to clean up nuclear waste. Long story short, bentonite clay is the real deal. When it comes in contact with a toxin, chemical, or heavy metal, the clay absorbs the toxin and releases its minerals for the body to use. In addition to being able to extract toxins, the clay contains nutrients including calcium, magnesium, silica, copper, iron, and potassium.

If you have a heart condition, have high blood pressure, are taking prescription medicine, or are pregnant, skip this bath. The Detoxifier bath uses bentonite clay, which may flush some minerals, vitamins, or electrolytes from the body along with the toxins. Therefore, do not take this bath after a heavy meal. Also, the clay may make the tub slippery, so be careful getting in and out of the bath.

Instructions:

Begin filling the tub with lukewarm water and add your stone(s). Once the stone is fully submerged, you can increase the water temperature to moderately hot if you'd like. (If you're using a gem elixir instead of a stone, add it once the tub is about a quarter full.) When the tub is a quarter full, add the clay, followed by the salt and baking soda, and mix them into the water using your hand. (To avoid lumps, mix the clay in a separate container with warm water before adding it to the bath.) Once the tub is three-quarters full, stop running the water and carefully get into the tub. Use any excess bentonite floating in the water as a body mask by gently rubbing it on your legs and arms. Soak for no more than 20 minutes, redistributing any sediment that settles on the bottom of the tub with your hand. If you feel sleepy, dizzy, or uncomfortable in any way, stand up slowly and exit the tub. Once you are finished with your bath, make certain to take a cool shower, as you want to rinse off any debris and any toxins that may have been pulled out of your body. Drain the tub and wipe it clean. Remove the stone. Rinse it under water to clean, and dry it with a soft cloth.

WHAT ARE BINAURAL BEATS?

Binaural beats are created by playing two loud tones (one in each ear) that are very close in frequency. Listeners to binaural beats "hear" a beat at a frequency equal to the difference between the frequencies of the applied tones. For example, if you play a 700 Hz tone in one ear and a 710 Hz tone in the other, your brain will create a binaural tone of 10 Hz. As the frequencies decrease, cognitive focus and alertness decrease, and you start moving into more meditative states, until you find yourself in a deep sleep. By listening regularly to different binaural beats optimized for different brain states, you may be able to induce relaxation, reduce stress and anxiety, and increase focus, concentration, motivation, confidence, and depth in meditation. There are also beats to strengthen your spiritual connection. While it's optimal to hear binaural beats using headphones, you can also experience their effect through speakers—and you'll want to while in the bath.

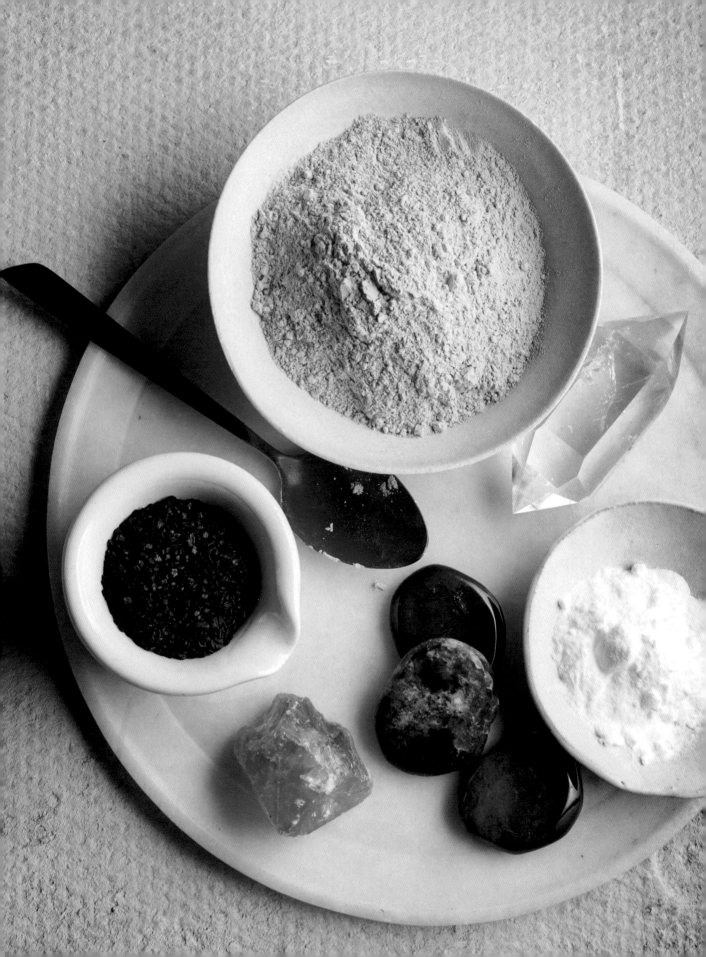

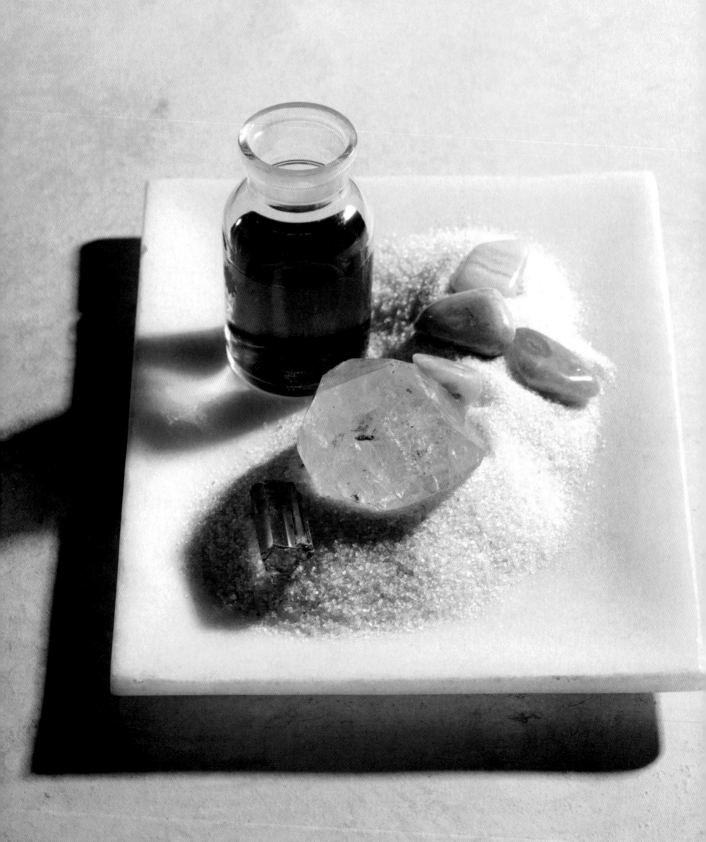

THE SPIRITUAL AWAKENER

This meditative bath incorporates the ancient ingredients frankincense, gold, and myrrh, which are referenced throughout the Bible and were used by the Greeks, Romans, Egyptians, and Chinese as medicine, incense, and perfume. Himalayan salt is known as white gold and contains the same eighty-four natural minerals and elements found in the human body. This peaceful, inspiring bath is designed to help you connect with the divine. To heighten the experience, try listening to classical music or binaural beats. While in the bath, you can also do a mini meditation: Hold a stone to your Heart chakra. Think of yourself connecting with a divine power. Imagine a light coming from the stone into your Heart chakra and running through every part of your body. Focus on your connection with your higher power, embracing and becoming one with the universe.

What you'll need:

- Suggested stone(s) and/or ½ cup gem elixir: blue lace agate, aquamarine, blue chalcedony, amethyst, herkimer diamond, sapphire, and/or onyx

- 6–8 drops myrrh, frankincense, geranium, rose, and/or sandalwood essential oil

- 1–2 cups Himalayan salt (preferred) or sea salt

- 2 tablespoons gold colloidal

Instructions:

Begin filling the tub with lukewarm water and add your stone(s). Once the stone is fully submerged, you can increase the water temperature to moderately hot if you'd like. (If you're using a gem elixir instead, add it once the tub is about a quarter full.) When the tub is a quarter full, add the essential oils. Add the salt followed by the gold colloidal and mix them into the water using your hand. Once the tub is three-quarters full, stop running the water and carefully get into the tub. Soak for up to 20 minutes or to your desired comfort level. Drain the tub and wipe it clean. Remove the stone and dry it with a soft cloth.

THE ILLUMINATING HYDRATOR

This luxurious update of Cleopatra's classic milk-and-honey bath hydrates and exfoliates. Pearl and gold brighten, illuminate, and recharge skin, leaving you glowing, soft, and supple. To heighten the experience, sip calming chamomile tea with honey during or after your bath.

What you'll need:

- Suggested stone(s) and/or ½ cup gem elixir: green moss agate, rose quartz, and/or aquamarine

- 2 cups whole milk

- ½ cup raw organic honey or organic honey

- 1 tablespoon gold colloidal

- ½ tablespoon pearl powder

- Essential oil for scent (optional): rose, lavender, geranium, and/or sandalwood

Power Ingredient: Raw Organic Honey

While you probably think of honey as something to sweeten your tea or spread on toast, raw honey can actually work wonders on your skin. Most honey found in grocery stores is processed and refined, killing its healing enzymes. Unprocessed or raw honey still contains gluconic acid, a mild alpha hydroxy acid that brightens the complexion, evening out skin tone and lightening scars and age spots. Most honey is also rich in minerals including iron, silica, copper, vitamin B, manganese, potassium, and calcium, which makes it excellent for skin. With its trace minerals, organic enzymes, and antioxidants, in addition to its antibacterial and antifungal properties, raw honey is a beauty go-to for all skin types.

Instructions:

Begin filling the tub with lukewarm water and add your stone(s). Once the stone is fully submerged, you can increase the water temperature to moderately hot if you'd like. (If you're using a gem elixir instead, add it once the tub is about a quarter full.) When the tub is a quarter full, add the milk and honey. (If you're using raw honey, spoon it into a coffee mug. Add boiling water and gently stir until melted. Raw honey is firm, and this is an easy way to emulsify it.)

Follow with the gold colloidal and pearl powder and mix them into the water using your hand. Once the tub is three-quarters full, stop running the water and carefully get into the tub. Soak for up to 20 minutes or to your desired comfort level. Drain the tub and wipe it clean. Remove the stone from the tub and dry it with a soft cloth.

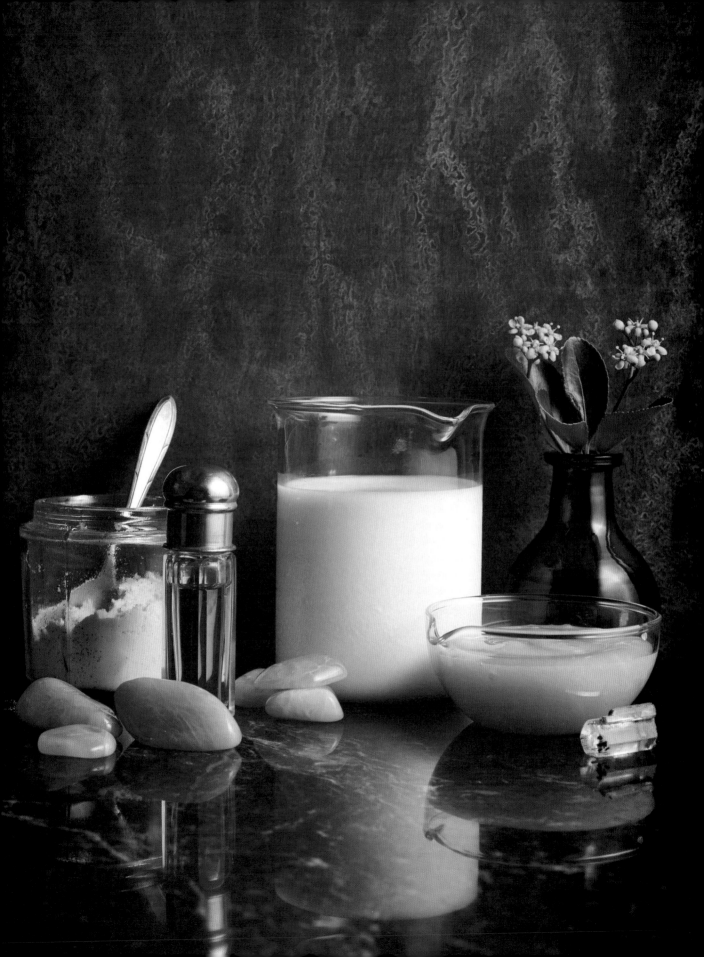

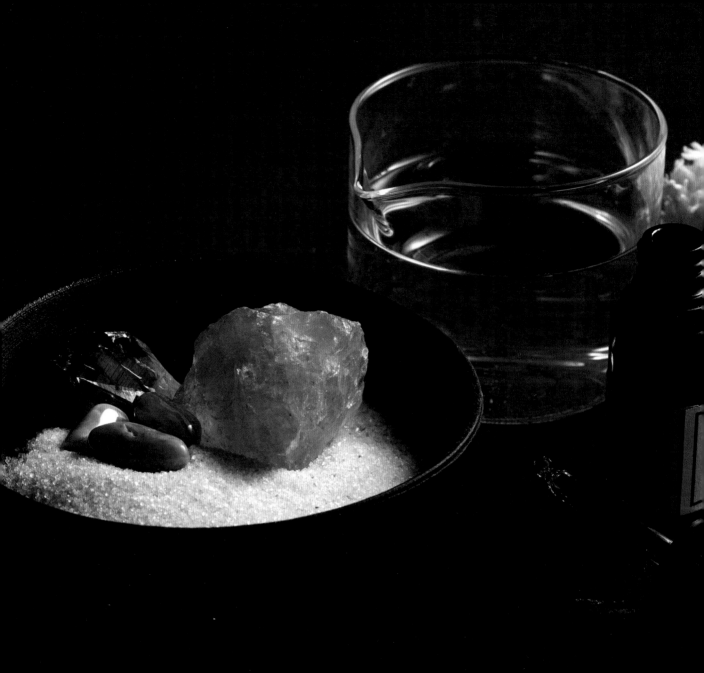

THE SERENITY CALMER

This bath is designed to calm all of your senses so you can relax and let go. Achieving a serene state can help lower stress and anxiety levels, leading to clearer thinking and a free flow of ideas. You're also likely to sleep better as a result. The essential oils and stones in this bath work to provide a sense of peace, love, and serenity. To heighten the experience, sip tea with rose hips, which are rich in vitamin C, vitamin E, and vitamin K, and take a deep breath and focus on your body's energy center—the heart. Research conducted by the HeartMath Institute, a nonprofit research and education organization offering prevention and intervention strategies for improved emotional health, suggests the heart to be approximately sixty times greater electrically than the brain and up to five thousand times stronger magnetically.

What you'll need:

- Suggested stone(s) and/or $\frac{1}{2}$ cup gemstone elixir: rose quartz, amethyst, blue lace agate, and/or aquamarine

- 6–8 drops rose essential oil (or try ylang-ylang, lavender, or chamomile)

- 1–2 cups Himalayan salt (preferred) or sea salt

- $\frac{1}{2}$ cup dried chamomile, lavender, or rose (optional)

Power Ingredient: Rose Essential Oil

Though known for its fragrance and supple petals, the rose's healing and antibacterial properties have been used for thousands of years in creams, emulsions, and soaps, while mildly astringent rose water can be used to cleanse dry and sensitive skin. A 2010 Chinese study compared rose essential oil to ten other oils and found that the rose oil not only exhibited one of the strongest bactericidal activities, but also just a small amount of it (.25 percent dilution) destroyed the bacteria responsible for acne after just five minutes. Another benefit of rose oil is it makes skin more permeable so that it's better able to absorb nutrients. On a metaphysical level, essential rose oil, which possesses a high vibrational frequency, is known to emanate love, purity, and wholeness while connecting the mind and body. Associated with the heart, rose oil is also said to help soothe stress and anxiety.

Instructions:

Begin filling the tub with lukewarm water and add your stone(s). Once the stone is fully submerged, you can increase the water temperature to moderately hot if you'd like. (If you're using a gem elixir instead, add it once the tub is about a quarter full.) When the tub is a quarter full, add the essential oil, salt, and dried flowers (if using) and mix them into the water using your hand. Once the tub is three-quarters full, stop running the water and carefully get into the tub. Soak for up to 20 minutes or to your desired comfort level. Drain the tub and wipe it clean. Remove the stone from the tub and dry it with a soft cloth.

THE COOLER

This bath is great during summer, in humid climates, or if you're feeling overheated. Blue lace agate, aquamarine, and amethyst are all cooling stones, and combined with the cucumber may help reduce swelling as well. The Cooler leaves the skin and body refreshed and awakened. For additional cooling, try drinking fresh aloe or cucumber water during or after your bath. *Note:* If you tend to be cold-blooded, this is most likely not the bath for you.

What you'll need:

- Suggested stone(s) and/or ½ cup gem elixir: blue lace agate, aquamarine, and/or amethyst

- 1 cup sea salt

- 2 tablespoons silver colloidal

- 1 sliced cucumber

Power Ingredient: Cucumber

Cucumbers are 95 percent water, so they're not only hydrating to eat, but also great for the skin. The anti-inflammatory compounds they contain help remove waste from the body and reduce skin irritation, according to the Cleveland Clinic. Preliminary research also suggests cucumbers promote antiwrinkling and antiaging activity. In addition, the juice of the cucumber will accelerate the healing of burns and wounds. Cucumbers are a great source of compounds that fight inflammation and aging, including cucurbitacins and cucumerin.

Instructions:

Begin filling the tub with lukewarm water and add your stone(s). Once the stone is fully submerged, you can increase the water temperature to moderately hot if you'd like. (If you're using a gem elixir instead, add it once the tub is about a quarter full.) When the tub is a quarter full, add the salt and silver colloidal and mix them into the water using your hand. Last, add the cucumber slices. Once the tub is three-quarters full, stop running the water and carefully get into the tub. Soak for 5 to 15 minutes (or as long as you are comfortable). This bath cools you rather quickly and is not recommended for an extended period of time. Drain the tub and wipe it clean. Remove the stone and dry it with a soft cloth.

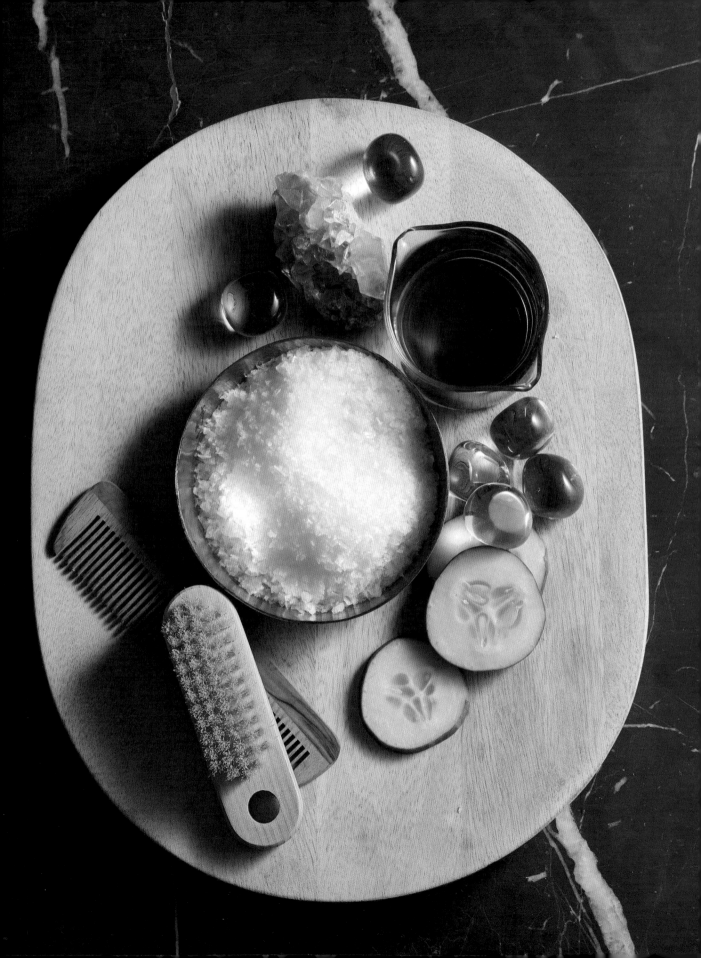

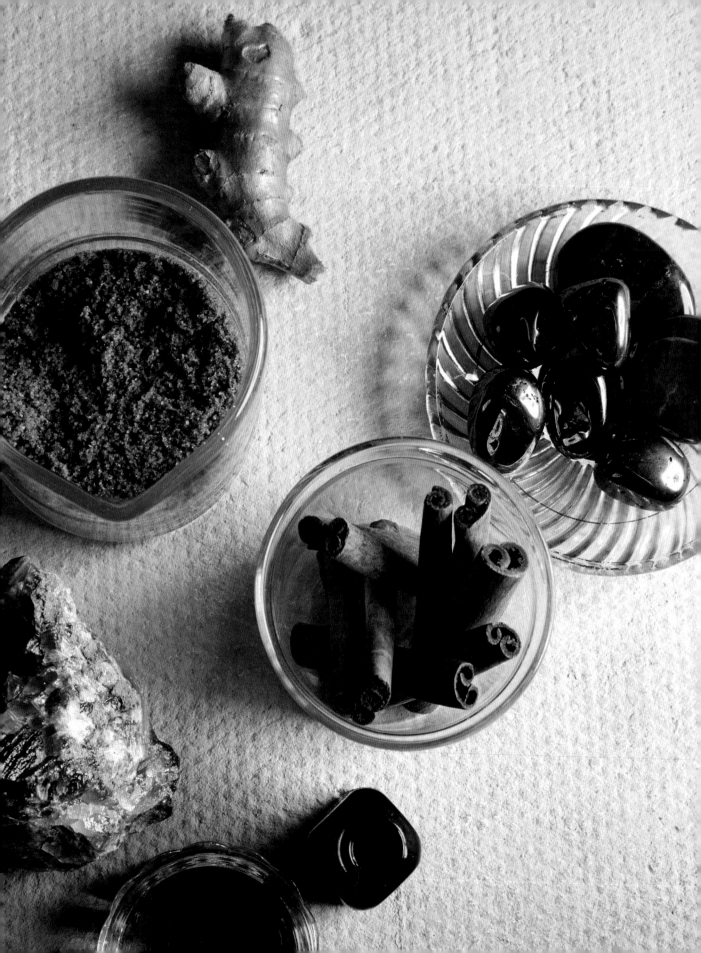

THE WARMING ENERGIZER

This bath stimulates and warms the body while lifting your spirit. Ginger and cinnamon can help raise your body temperature and are enhanced when combined with warming and energizing stones like carnelian, rose quartz, or hematite. It's perfect for a winter day or when you are feeling a touch under the weather. To heighten the experience, sip warm water or ginger tea with lemon during or after the bath. *Note*: If you are warm-blooded, this is most likely not the bath for you.

What you'll need:

♦ Suggested stone(s) and/or ½ cup gem elixir: rose quartz, ruby, carnelian, red jasper, bloodstone, and/or hematite

♦ 1 cup sea salt or red Hawaiian sea salt

♦ 1 tablespoon gold colloidal

♦ ¼ cup sliced ginger root

♦ 2 cinnamon sticks

♦ 2 drops sweet orange essential oil (optional)

Power Ingredient: Ginger

Ginger is warming on a cold day, and it can help promote healthy sweating, which is why your doctor may suggest drinking hot water with ginger if you have a cold or the flu. Both ingesting ginger and applying it topically may have major antiaging benefits—it contains around forty antioxidant properties that protect against aging. In addition, ginger has anti-inflammatory properties, so adding ginger oil to your bath can help relieve muscle and joint aches.

Instructions:

Begin filling the tub with lukewarm water and add your stone(s). Once the stone is fully submerged, you can increase the water temperature to moderately hot if you'd like. (If you're using a gem elixir instead, add it once the tub is about a quarter full.) When the tub is a quarter full, add the salt, gold colloidal, ginger, cinnamon, and essential oil (if using) and mix them into the water using your hand. Once the tub is three-quarters full, stop running the water and carefully get into the tub. Soak for up to 20 minutes or to your desired comfort level. Drain the tub and wipe it clean. Remove the stone and dry it with a soft cloth.

THE CLEARING BATH

This bath was created to help clear your mind, body, and the aura or energy field that surrounds you. As we are energetic beings, it is important to take time to balance and clear our energy field, allowing for a more lucid state. The bath incorporates a colloidal blend of silver, gold, and copper believed to aid in balancing body, mind, and spirit. When taking this bath, imagine a peaceful white light gently sweeping through you, cleansing and renewing every cell of your body.

What you'll need:

- Suggested stone(s) and/or ½ cup gem elixir: clear quartz, Herkimer diamond, and/or diamond
- 1 cup Himalayan salt or sea salt
- ½ teaspoon clear quartz powder (optional)
- 2 tablespoons gold colloidal, or 1 tablespoon gold colloidal plus 1 tablespoon silver colloidal and 1 tablespoon copper colloidal

Power Ingredient: Himalayan Crystal Salt

The purest salt on earth, Himalayan crystal salt gets it natural pink color from its iron content. For centuries, Himalayan salt has been used for protection and purification, since it is believed to have grounding, calming, and clarifying properties. Like crystals and gemstones, Himalayan salt is formed over millions of years under tectonic pressure, free of exposure to toxins and impurities. Himalayan salt not only contains eighty-four minerals and elements found in the human body, but it also has a unique crystalline structure that allows it to store vibrational energy. The minerals and trace elements in the salt exist in colloidal form, making it easy for cells to absorb them.

Instructions:

Begin filling the tub with lukewarm water and add your stone(s). Once the stone is fully submerged, you can increase the water temperature to moderately hot if you'd like. (If you're using a gem elixir instead, add it once the tub is about a quarter full.) When the tub is a quarter full, add the salt, quartz powder (if using), and the colloidals and mix them into the water using your hand. Once the tub is three-quarters full, stop running the water and carefully get into the tub. Soak for up to 20 minutes or to your desired comfort level. Drain the tub and wipe it clean. Remove the stone and dry it with a soft cloth.

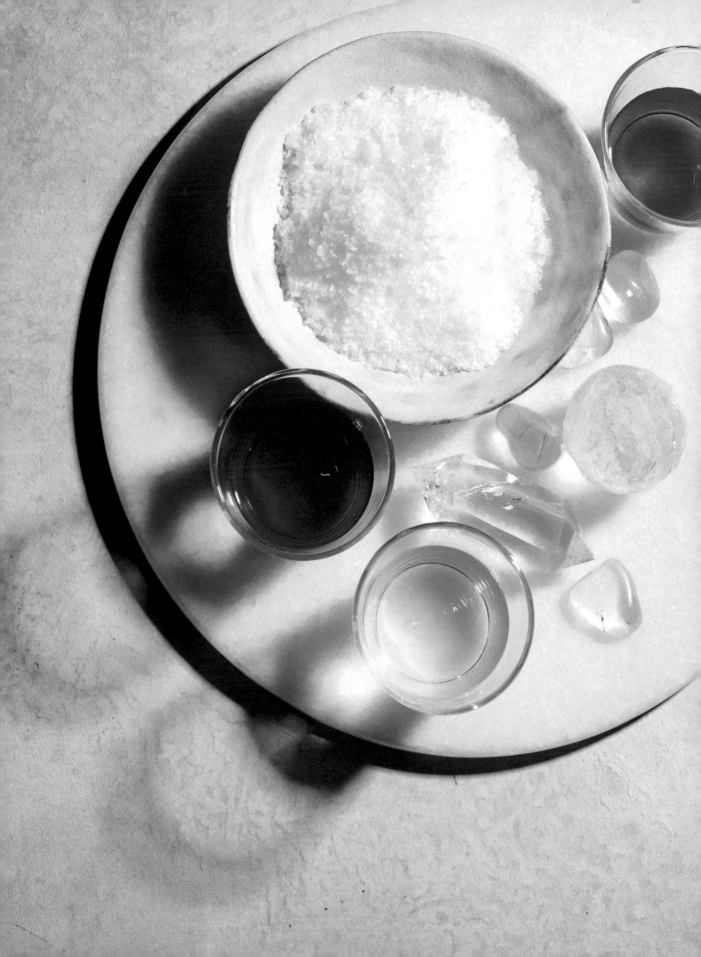

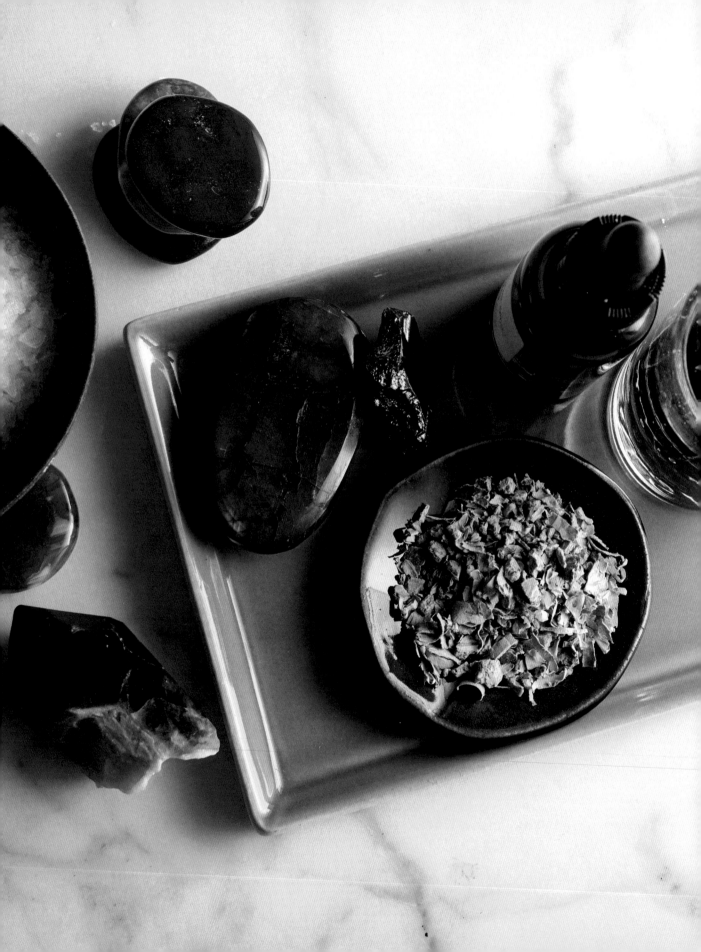

THE GROUNDING BATH

This is the perfect bath for those times when you could use a little help feeling centered, rooted, and stable. Birch and a combination of green and dark stones like moss agate and hematite connect you with the earth, helping you in feeling grounded. Drinking licorice or anise tea during or after the bath will further increase your sense of rootedness, as will practicing this meditation: Take one of the stones in the bath and place it under one of your feet, keeping your feet flat against the tub. Visualize yourself as a tree with roots growing deep into the ground and think or say "I am rooted, centered, and grounded" until you begin to feel a wholeness or oneness within your body.

What you'll need:

- Green stone(s) and/or ¼ cup gem elixir: moss agate and/or jade
- Dark stone(s) and/or ¼ cup gem elixir: hematite, smoky quartz, and/or black tourmaline
- 1 cup sea salt
- 2 teaspoons gold colloidal
- 6–8 drops cedarwood, spruce, juniper, white fir, or angelica essential oil
- ½ cup birch wood chips (optional)

Power Ingredient: Birch

The birch tree is sometimes referred to as the "tree of life" because of its anti-inflammatory properties—courtesy of betulinic acid—which are helpful in treating conditions like arthritis, high cholesterol, heart and kidney edema, and cystitis. Birch also possesses strong astringent properties, which make it great for treating skin conditions like eczema and dermatitis. Unlike other tree oils, birch doesn't have a woody aroma. Instead, it smells minty, like wintergreen. Its properties and uses are also very similar to wintergreen's; both contain a natural form of methyl salicylate, a compound known for soothing achy muscles and joints. Emotionally, it's said to be the oil of support, helping you find your own inner strength, rooting you and allowing you to seek, find, and receive support in new ways. It may also help when you're feeling scattered, overwhelmed, or lacking connection with others.

Instructions:

Begin filling the tub with lukewarm water and add your stones. Once the stones are fully submerged, you can increase the water temperature to moderately hot if you'd like. (If you're using gem elixirs instead, add them once the tub is about a quarter full.) When the tub is a quarter full, add the salt, gold colloidal, essential oil, and wood chips and mix them into the water using your hand. Once the tub is three-quarters full, stop running the water and carefully get into the tub. Soak for up to 20 minutes or to your desired comfort level. Drain the tub and wipe it clean. Remove the stones and dry them with a soft cloth.

FOOTBATHS

While you may not have time every day for a relaxing soak in the tub, you can always end your day with a ten-minute foot soak to reap the benefits of a gemstone-infused bath without the time commitment.

Footbaths have long been an important tool for detoxifying, cleansing, and relaxing. In Japan, public footbaths where locals congregate to soak their feet and legs publicly, called *ashiyu*, can be found on street corners in towns with hot springs. In fact, footbaths are so popular in the country that they have been installed in high-speed bullet trains so passengers can sit, four at a time, with their feet in the baths, before retiring to an "after-bath lounge car" for locally brewed sake. Similarly, Traditional Chinese Medicine recommends daily footbaths that promote blood circulation. The reason so many spas in the western hemisphere have adopted footbaths as a pretreatment ritual is that a foot soak soothes aching muscles, hydrates skin, and relieves aches and pains associated with wearing fashionable high heels for hours on end. Plus, letting your feet sit in a bath can help reduce swelling and prevent bacteria from settling into blisters and cuts.

Simply soaking your feet in warm water is surprisingly effective. Six meridians (liver, gallbladder, kidney, spleen, and stomach) reach the feet, each of which has more than sixty acupuncture points. Therefore, soaking feet in hot water activates blood and energy throughout the body. Ideally, you want to submerge your feet and calves in water—you can sit on the side of a tub, placing your feet inside, or use a deep metal washbasin in which you can submerge your feet while sitting in your favorite chair. (If the weather's nice, you can do this outdoors while enjoying the sunset.)

Adding your favorite gemstone to the water can help bring desired results, whether you use amethyst to help with feelings of grief or guilt, aquamarine to improve concentration, clear quartz to bring clarity and open the senses, or any of the stones mentioned in chapter 3. But you can further personalize your footbath by adding fresh flowers or a few drops of essential oil. Some good choices for tired feet are *juniper berry oil*, which alleviates muscle aches, including those caused by arthritis; *lavender oil*, which is a natural pain reliever, optimal for sore muscles and joints; *rosemary oil*, which helps soothe tired muscles and has antiseptic properties; and *wintergreen oil*, which assists with pain and swelling and has a cooling sensation that is pleasurable on tired feet. You can also add a cup of *Epsom salts*, a compound that can help flush toxins and heavy metals from your skin's cells, reduce inflammation, increase circulation, and ease muscle cramps and joint pain.

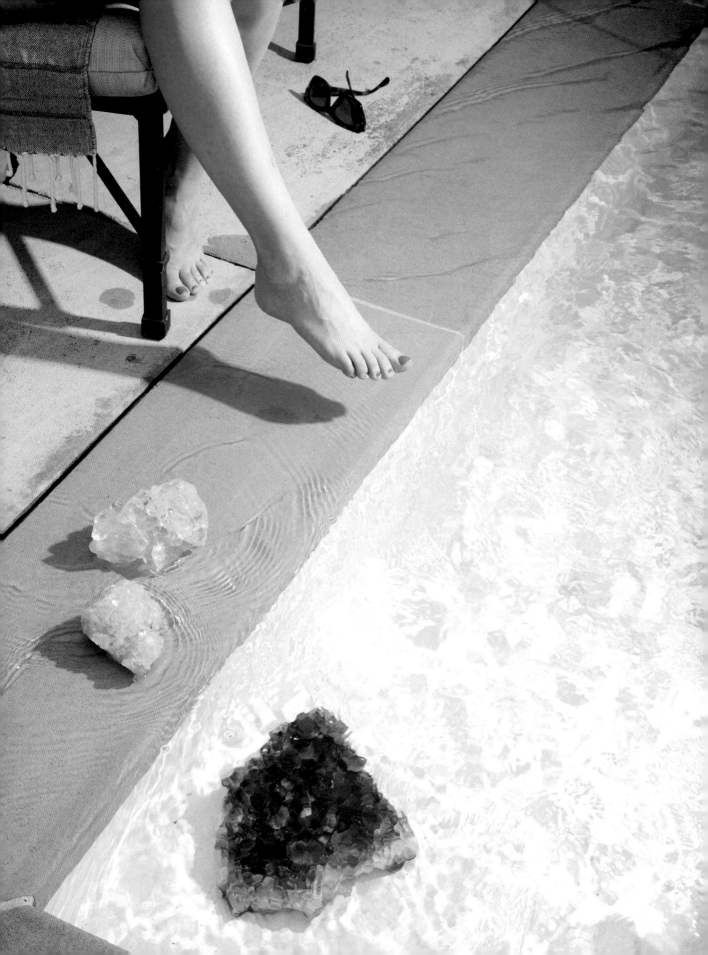

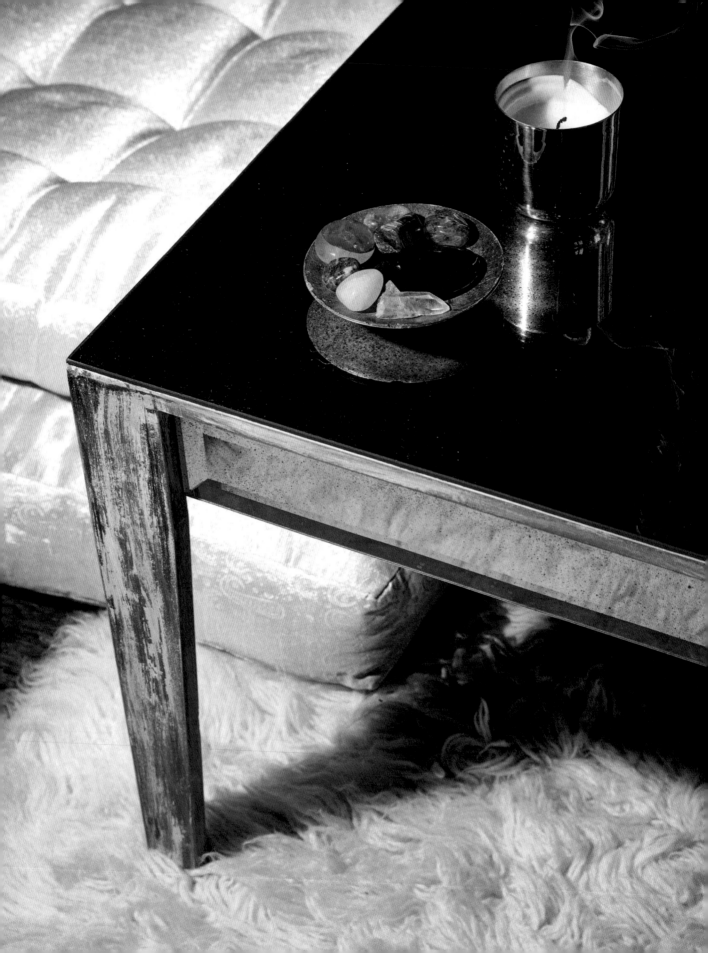

7

LAYING OF STONES

HEAD-TO-TOE ENERGY FLOW

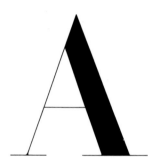s I hope you've seen for yourself by now, the ability of crystals and gemstones to harmonize and balance the body while soothing the mind and tapping into the potential of the spirit is a miraculous gift from nature. You now have an arsenal of naturally beautiful, restorative tools at your disposal the next time you're feeling unfocused, exhausted, or overwhelmed. (Talk about a gift that keeps on giving!)

In this chapter, I want to introduce you to another ritual, laying of stones, which has been practiced for thousands of years. The ritual involves placing stones at points on the body that correspond to the chakras, or energy centers. This is known as "chakra clearing," "chakra opening," or "chakra balancing." Balancing your chakras through the laying of stones not only keeps both blood and energy flowing throughout the body, but it also infuses the body with the energy of the gemstones, supporting its natural healing process. The ritual comes to us in the present day through the teachings of Indian Vedic texts written more than five thousand years ago. Today, healers lay stones to relieve stress, particularly during times of change; improve self-esteem; sharpen concentration; aid in creative and personal growth; and promote inner harmony and balance.

I experienced the power of a chakra opening through the laying of stones shortly after my father passed away suddenly in 2011. I felt deeply off center and out of balance. My

Heart chakra energy was low, which at first I *sensed* more than rationally knew. What I didn't realize at the time is that when one or more of your chakra energies is running low, it can affect all aspects of your life, from the free flow of thoughts and ideas to relationships, health, and spiritual connection. I was familiar with chakra balancing from the själ facial, which seeks to generally align the body's energy as part of the treatment. During the facial, I had always responded most powerfully to the rose quartz placed on my Heart chakra.

After my father passed, I found myself thinking about the Heart chakra more and more. One evening, I set aside some quiet time by myself. After setting an intention, "Please allow my Heart to open," which I repeated several times, I lay down and placed a pink rose quartz and a green malachite on my Heart chakra. I visualized my heart expanding, making room for love and acceptance. As I let go, I felt a subtle yet powerful surge of energy around my heart that blanketed me with warmth as it expanded outward like the sun's rays. Afterward, I felt at peace, and the heaviness in my heart dissipated. The hurt and sadness that had engulfed me since my dad was first diagnosed with cancer had softened its grip on my heart, so I could begin to heal. In time, I felt ready to engage with the world again, to explore new ideas and places, and to get back to living and loving fully and unconditionally.

As with any successful healing or opening, having the right tools on hand is key. In this case, crystals and gemstones are *the* keys to the kingdom. And laying the stones couldn't be simpler: you simply place one or more gemstones or crystals of a color that corresponds to one of the seven chakra points on or near that point, then leave them there for a period of time to help open the chakras. Don't let the simplicity of the ritual fool you; I find it incredibly effective for moving stagnant energy. If you don't experience movement, small clear quartz apexes placed strategically around your body can assist in amplifying another stone's energy.

You may, as I did, feel your chakras open after just one clearing session. But if you don't, keep at it. Moving energy that has been stagnant for months or even years is a process, a practice, and a slow build. As with exercise, you've got to keep at it to see and feel the changes in energy flow, which at times can be subtle.

How long should you set aside to perform the laying-of-stones rituals outlined in this chapter? I suggest at least fifteen to twenty minutes, although leaving them on longer is fine. If you feel uncomfortable at any point remove the stone, cleanse it, and try again at another time. After the first week, during which you'll start slowly by laying just one stone each day on a corresponding chakra point, aim for three sessions a week. Remember, clearing out the residue from physical, emotional, mental, and spiritual imbalances can lead to positive opportunities personally, professionally, and spiritually, so the time you invest in yourself can yield valuable dividends.

THE SEVEN CHAKRAS

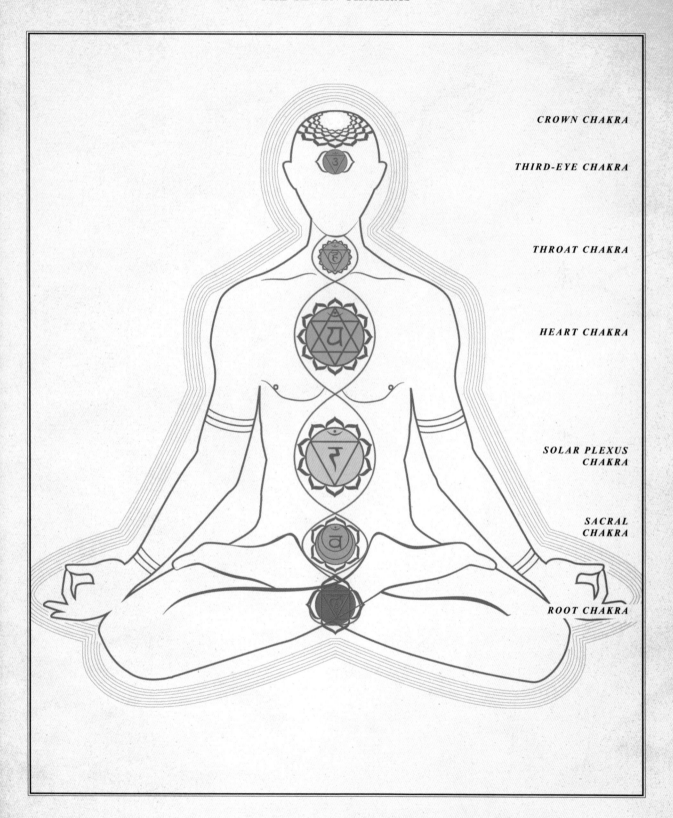

CROWN CHAKRA

THIRD-EYE CHAKRA

THROAT CHAKRA

HEART CHAKRA

SOLAR PLEXUS
CHAKRA

SACRAL
CHAKRA

ROOT CHAKRA

LAY IT ON: THE STONE-CHAKRA CONNECTION

	COLOR ASSOCIATION	LOCATION	WHEN IT'S LOW	
Root or Base Chakra *Represents passion and the feeling of being grounded*	Red	Base of the spine	You may feel weak, tired, or unmotivated; experience lower-back or leg pain or immune-system disorders; or go into survival mode.	
Sacral Chakra *Represents creativity and your ability to accept others*	Orange	Two inches below the navel	You may feel confused, overly dependent on others, frustrated, or lacking motivation, and you may experience swelling or low levels of hormones.	
Solar Plexus Chakra *Represents intellect and how you see yourself in the world*	Yellow	Upper abdomen	You may feel controlling, fearful, lack self-confidence, or an inability to experience emotions. You may experience digestive problems.	
Heart Chakra *Represents your ability to love unconditionally and accept others*	Green	Center of chest	You may feel stressed, anxious, jealous, or bitter, and you may experience high or low blood pressure, high or low heart rate, or lumps or cysts in your breasts.	
Throat Chakra *Represents communication and self-expression*	Blue	Throat	You may feel a lack of ability to express yourself in a positive manner or at a loss for words, and you may experience stuttering, feelings of isolation or being misunderstood, sore throat, tight jaw, or stiff neck.	
Third Eye or Brow Chakra *Represents understanding and your ability to focus on and see the big picture*	Indigo	Between the eyes on the forehead	You may experience a foggy brain, overactive mind, stiff neck, or inflexibility.	
Crown Chakra *Represents divine inspiration*	Violet	Top of the head	You may feel clumsy, uncoordinated, uninspired, out of step, unsure of who you are or why you exist, or rigid in your thinking.	

Each chakra is associated with a particular location of the body and a particular color. Each chakra also has its own particular role in optimal health and well-being.

	WHEN IT'S OPEN	DO THIS	STONES
	You will feel "at home" in your body, empowered, and full of life.	Place a *red* stone between your thighs near the groin and think of the color red—warmth, your foundation, core, family (if this feels stable), or your passion.	Red jasper, ruby, and bloodstone
	You'll feel flexible in both body and mind, creative, playful, and open.	Place an *orange* stone above the pelvic bone, think of the color orange, and think of yourself as a creative being.	Carnelian, dark or brown citrine, orange aventurine, orange calcite, and tangerine quartz
	You may release the need to control, and be open to new ideas, suggestions, emotions, happiness, and joy. You may experience robust digestion.	Place a *yellow* stone two inches above your belly button, think of the color yellow or a sunny day, and think of your power center and your ability to manifest.	Citrine and amber
	You may feel more relaxed, accepting, open to new relationships, and able to sustain balanced relationships. You may feel love and forgiveness.	Place a *green* or *pink* stone on your breastbone, think of the colors pink and green, and think of soothing, mending, opening your heart. (Rose quartz is known for nurturing and restructuring the emotional centers of the heart. Think of the green as soothing and healing the heart). Let any anger go.	For green: malachite, green tourmaline, green moss agate, emerald, and aventurine; for pink: rose quartz, ruby, rhodochrosite, and pink tourmaline; or for pink and green: watermelon tourmaline
	You may feel more expressive, communicative, and true to yourself, and you may experience healthier mouth, gums, teeth, and nasal passages.	Place a *blue* stone on the larynx, think of the color blue, and think of clear communication, positive speech, and power in your words.	Blue sapphire, sodalite, lapis lazuli, aquamarine, and turquoise
	You may experience a clearer mind, an enhanced ability to problem solve, a greater intuition, and the ability to understand and focus.	Place a *purple* stone between the brows (the Third Eye is a calming spot), think of the color purple, and focus on your intuition and clarity.	Amethyst, lapis, and iolite
	You may feel more flexible, understanding of the ebb and flow of life, unruffled by setbacks, and have a clearer ability to see things as they are.	Place a *clear* or *violet* stone above your head, think of a white light, and think of your connection with the divine, God, and/or spirit.	Clear quartz and light amethyst

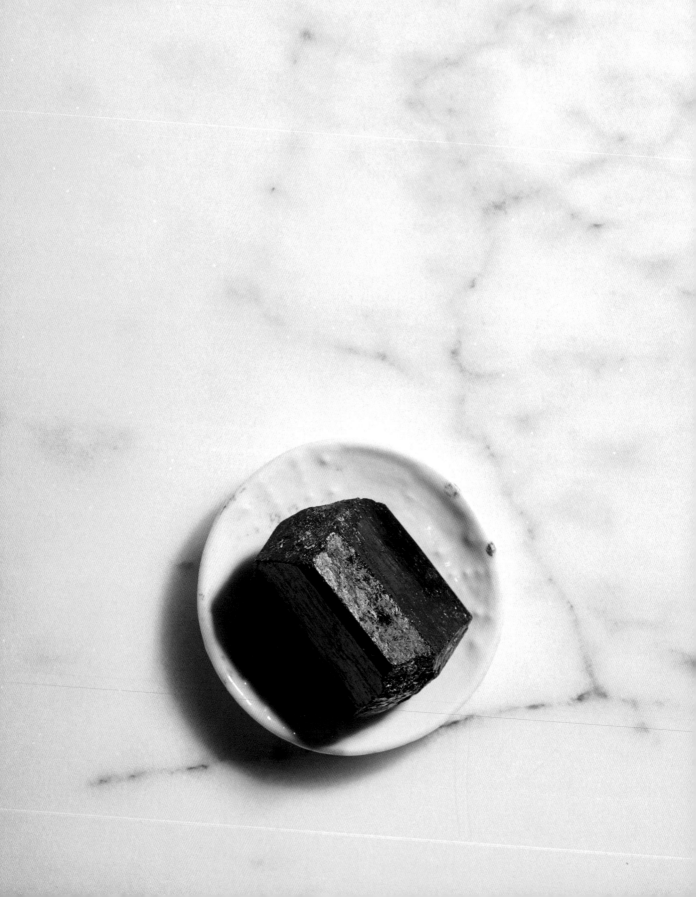

*As with any treatment or ritual, start slowly
and build gradually. Give your body time to
receive each stone's energy and learn how it feels
to stimulate and open each energy center.*

There are a few things to do before you begin any of the rituals: Take the time to cleanse and charge your stones first (see "Bringing Home Your Crystals and Gems," page 64). Remember to switch off your phone so you can enjoy the healing benefits of the ritual without any interruptions. (Even most of the important calls and texts can wait twenty minutes!) Play peaceful music to set the tone. Keep a notebook nearby so that afterward you can jot down any feelings or sensations you experience. And remember to drink plenty of distilled water as you detoxify!

There are also a few tools I like to use to complement and enhance any laying-of-stones ritual. The first helps keep me grounded, particularly when clearing the Third Eye or Crown chakras, while the second and third amplify the energy of any stone, maximizing my time on the table, bed, or couch.

The first tool is a dark stone placed beneath the heel of each foot. While you ultimately want to clear all of your chakras, you also want to make sure that you ground yourself while doing so, as you are of the earth and need to accomplish things on it (which is hard to do if you are feeling spaced-out and light-headed). Any dark stone—from black tourmaline or hematite to smoky quartz or obsidian—will do the trick.

The second tool is a purple plate, placed on the surface on which you are lying, to amplify energy. (For more on purple plates, see "A Tool Named for Tesla," page 68.) I always like to place a Tesla plate below my feet, under my hips, or between my heart and shoulders, depending on my areas of focus.

The third tool is an amethyst biomat. Amethyst has been called "nature's tranquilizer" by many health practitioners because of its effectiveness in relaxing the mind *and* the nervous system. Although I have had some of my most transformative healing sessions lying on top of an amethyst biomat, they are expensive (full-size ones run $1,500 and up). That said, biomats are Food and Drug Administration–licensed medical devices approved to treat minor muscle and joint pain as well as minor sprains and muscular back pain. You may also find that they improve sleep, reduce inflammation, and support the immune system, though the FDA does not license them for these purposes.

CHAKRA CLEARING IN THREE PARTS

As with any treatment or ritual, it's always wise to start slowly and build gradually. This gives your body time to receive each stone's energy and you time to learn how it feels to stimulate and open each energy center. Because of this, I think it makes sense to introduce chakra clearing through laying of stones into your life in three parts. In part 1, you'll take a week to lay a different-colored stone each day on a corresponding chakra point for fifteen to twenty minutes. In part 2, you'll practice opening all seven chakras simultaneously. In part 3, which I call "laying-of-stones 2.0," you'll witness the power of crystals and gemstones to strengthen the body as well as the mind-spirit connection.

PART 1
A CHAKRA A DAY

Since balancing the chakras can be a powerful experience, you'll want to gradually work your way up to a full-body clearing. And since there are seven chakras, you can devote one day to each chakra for the first week. On Monday, start at the Root and lay a single red stone there for twenty minutes. On Tuesday, lay a yellow stone on the Solar Plexus. Work your way up the chakras each following day, choosing an appropriate stone from "Lay It On" (pages 138–39), until you reach the Crown on Sunday. By focusing on one chakra at a time, you'll get a sense of how it feels to clear or move energy from a particular point. Lie still and bring your focus to your body. Stay open to any pulsations, tingling, or warmth you may feel. Also, be open to any release of emotions that may need to be cleared.

CLEAR QUARTZ ENERGY FLOW

I've said it before, but I can't stress enough how important it is to have plenty of clear quartz apexes (stones with one pointed end) on hand. They work like magnets to balance, increase, or clear energy, depending on which way you face the points. It's as easy as that! You can use the clear quartz apexes to enhance any of the laying-of-stones rituals, or try one of the following exercises on its own.

After each twenty-minute session, ask yourself, "How did this stone affect my body?" The more you perform these rituals, the more in tune you'll be with how the energy feels and the synergy between you and the stones.

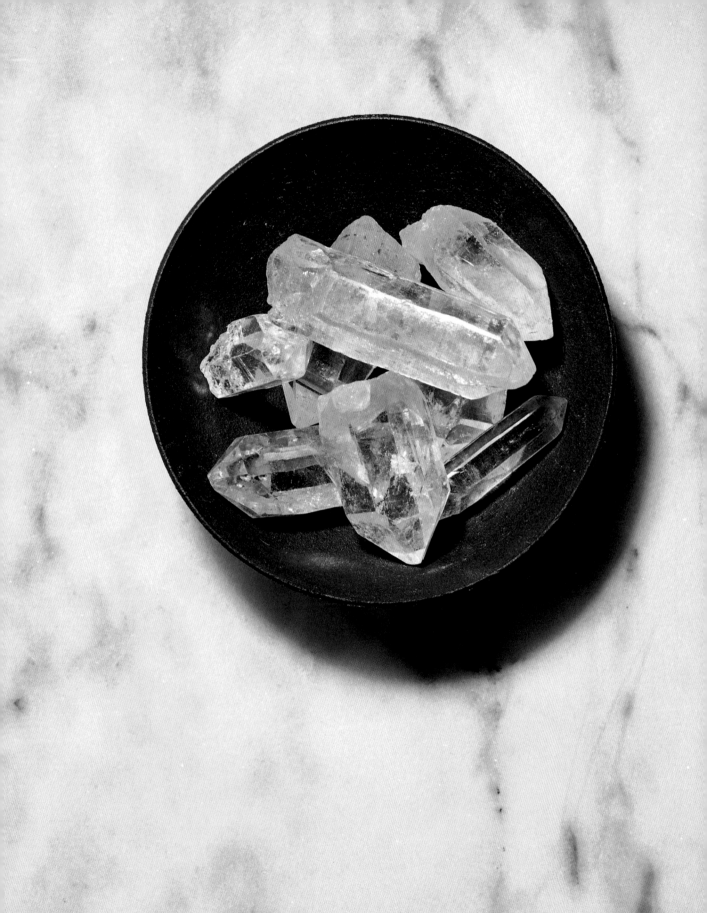

CREATING A CIRCUIT

Place a clear quartz apex or point in the palm of each hand. Point the one in the left hand toward your body (energy coming in). The one in the right hand should point outward or away from your body (energy going out). This creates a circle or wheel of energy, producing a balancing effect throughout the body. Hold the apexes in place for fifteen to twenty minutes and breathe. This exercise can be done alone or in addition to any treatment.

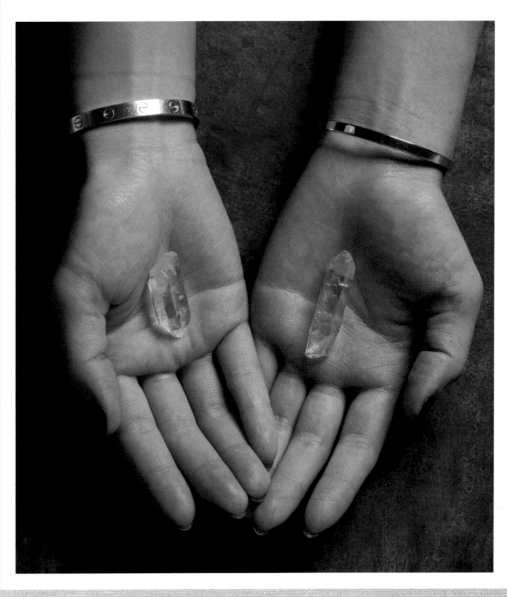

PART 2

A FULL-BODY CHAKRA OPENING

Once you've familiarized yourself with how the various-hued stones correspond to your chakra points, you can try laying a stone on each point simultaneously. Lie down on a comfortable surface and place each colored stone on the corresponding chakra point; make sure to place dark stones beneath each foot, behind knees, or behind ankles for grounding. Start by visualizing a warm grounding energy moving up from your Root or Base to your Sacral with a feeling of creativity; then to the Solar Plexus for self-empowerment; then to the Heart, which brings love, openness, and acceptance; then to your Throat for communication and your Third Eye for intuition and guidance; and then ultimately bringing this energy to the Crown for divine connection. The energy then travels back down to the Root or Base, continuing to bring energy up and through the body, creating a wheel of light or wheel of life. Immerse yourself in the energy.

> ### INCREASING OR CLEARING ENERGY
>
> To enhance energy or energize the body, you'll need nine clear quartz apexes. Lie down and lay the apexes so they encircle the body with apexes facing inward (toward the body) in the following places: below each foot, outside each knee, on each side of the torso, above each shoulder, and above the top of the head. For a serious energy boost and grounding experience, place hematite stones on all seven chakras after laying the quartz apexes in place. To clear energy, follow the above steps but point the quartz apexes outward, away from the body.

Just remember that at the end of the full-body session, you need to "close" the chakras one by one: Start by visualizing a white light coming down over and into the Crown chakra. Bring the light down through the chakras to the Root chakra. Then begin to close each chakra by imagining a shield of white light over each, starting with the Root and working your way up through each chakra. Envision yourself in a pyramid or blanket of white light with mirrors on the outside of the pyramid all around, facing outward. Anything coming at you will be reflected outward with love and light.

If you feel that a chakra may need additional balancing or clearing, you may place the stone or stones that correspond with that chakra on *all* of the chakra points along your body, aligning all chakras with the same stone (e.g., if you feel your Heart chakra needs additional balancing, you would place nurturing rose quartz on every chakra).

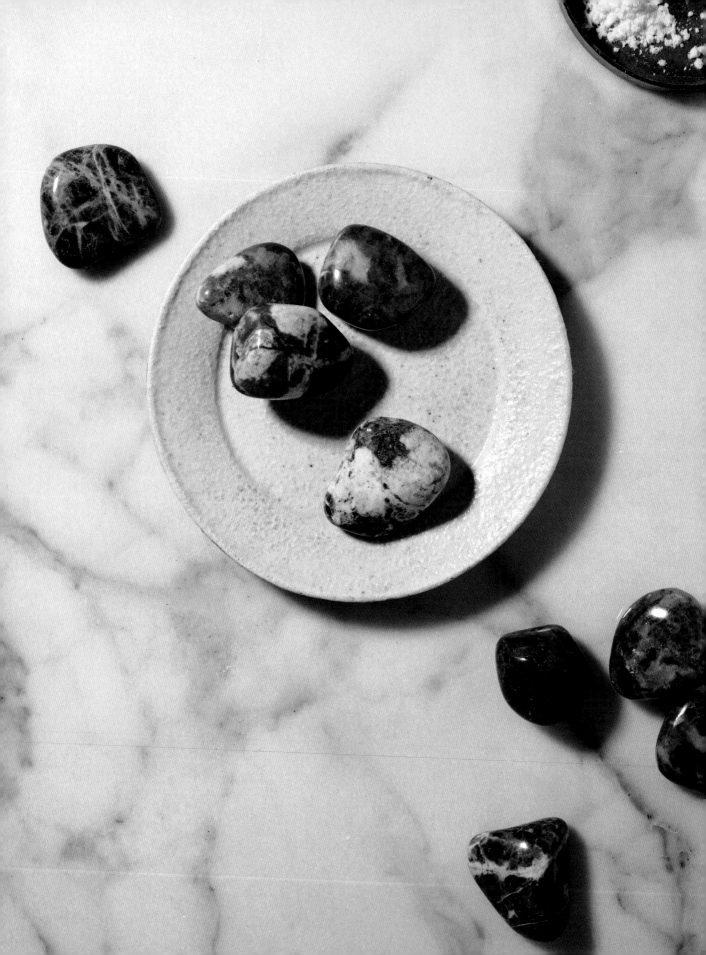

PART 3
RITUALS FOR BODY, MIND, AND SPIRIT

Ready to take things to the next level? These rituals focus on detoxifying the lymphatic system, clearing the heart through forgiveness, and establishing a clear connection between the mind and the spirit. For some of these rituals, you will need a stone other than the ones listed in "The Elemental Ten" from chapter 3 (see page 40). All rituals should be performed for at least twenty minutes.

LYMPHATIC SYSTEM DETOXIFICATION (RENEWED ENERGY)

Polluted air, pesticide-treated and genetically modified food, and impure water can cause an increase of metabolic waste in the body that may be toxic. As a result, you may feel tired, moody, and low in energy. This ritual can help to detoxify the lymphatic system so energy can flow freely through it. Keep in mind that at first you may not feel great when you're detoxing, because you're bringing your body, which gets used to the status quo of not feeling so well, back to its pure state.

1. Lie down and place ten pieces of sodalite on the following locations: one on the Third Eye chakra, two on either side of the neck below the jawbone, one on the Throat chakra, one on the Heart chakra (on the breastbone), one under each armpit, one on the Root chakra (on the groin), and one on each knee. Try adding a pinch of organic cream of tartar under the tongue to help cleanse the lymph system.

2. Think of your body as a clear tube with energy flowing in and out. Imagine a white light flowing through the tube up and down like the traffic on a two-way street.

3. Place a pinch of organic cream of tartar under your tongue to help cleanse the lymph system. Afterward, drink a cup of green tea to flush away any remaining toxins.

HEART
(FORGIVENESS AND PEACE)

This ritual can be transformative if you're holding on to emotional baggage, sadness, resentment, and feel you need more work on your heart than a basic chakra clearing offers. To heal, you need to forgive and let go of negative thoughts so that you can feel unconditional love for yourself and others. When you place pink and green stones on the Heart chakra, you move out stale energy while the stones soothe and infuse your heart with warmth and love. Afterward, the heart should feel joyful, peaceful, and at ease in the body—not strangled or overwhelmed. The more you open your heart, the more clearly you see what's holding you back and what you *should* be doing in your life.

1. Lie down and place the following stones on your breastbone: malachite (to open emotional issues), rose quartz (to heal any damage done), carnelian (to help bring oxygen to the heart area), and green tourmaline or watermelon tourmaline (for regeneration).

2. Place four clear quartz apexes around the stones, with the points facing the Heart.

3. Breathe deeply into your Heart. Think to yourself, "As I open up my heart, I ask for peace and forgiveness." Allow yourself to feel love, envisioning a beautiful light in your heart gently expanding, experiencing waves of peace, and allowing yourself to let go of any anger or sadness that may be deep within.

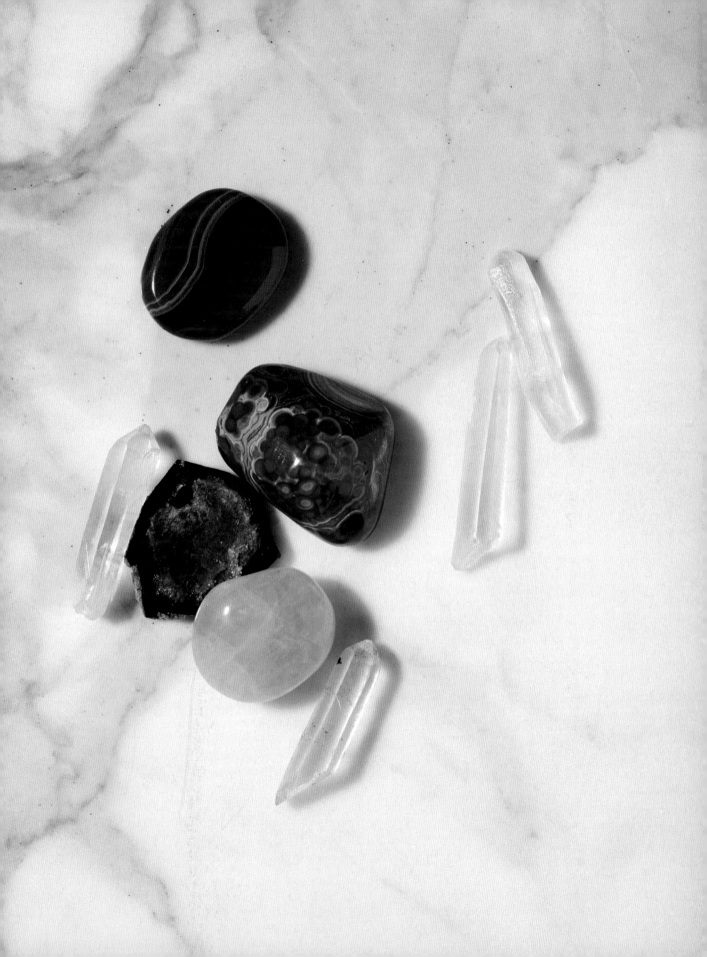

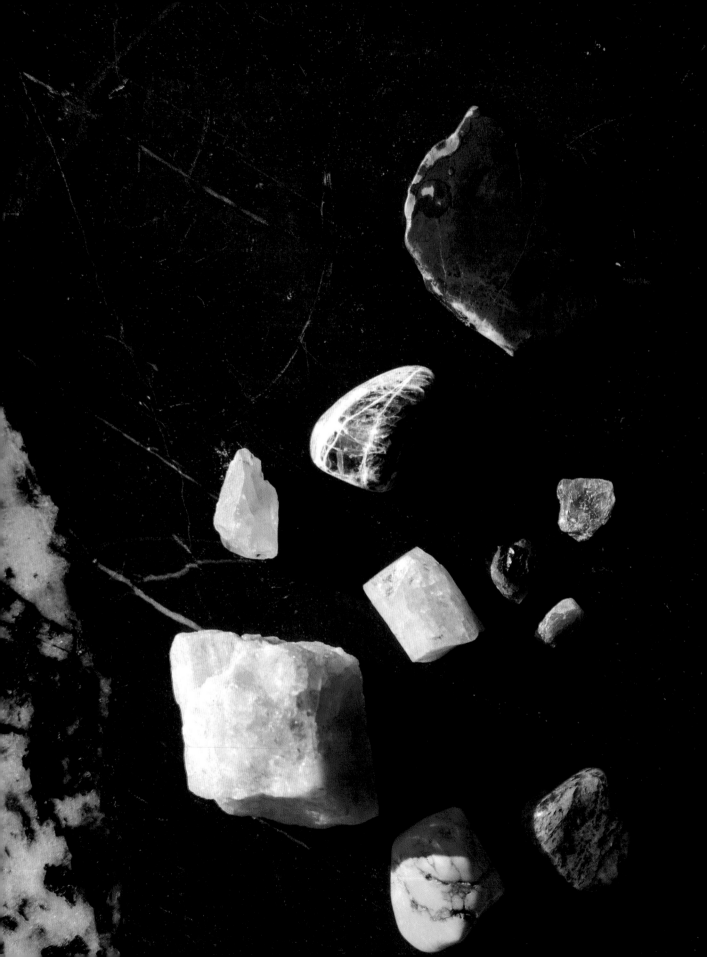

MIND AND SPIRIT
(CLEARING OLD THOUGHT PATTERNS)

What we think as well as feel transfers to our physical body, which is why it's important to clear old thought patterns and establish a direct link between our physical and spiritual selves.

1. Lie down and place any blue stone (suggested: aquamarine, sodalite, lapis lazuli, or blue lace agate) on the Throat chakra.

2. Place a sapphire or lapis lazuli on the Third Eye chakra.

3. Place an amethyst just above the Third Eye chakra.

4. Place a clear quartz two inches above your head (if the stone has a natural apex, point it away from the head.)

5. Place a dark grounding stone, such as tourmaline or hematite, on the groin, the hips, and the Root chakra.

6. Breathe deeply into your lower body, focusing on your belly and sacrum. Think to yourself, "All negative thought patterns are being cleared away."

YOU HAVE CHAKRA POINTS *WHERE?*

While I was familiar with the seven chakra points before I ever thought to enhance, move, and clear their energy with gemstones and crystals, I was surprised to learn that hands and feet also contain chakra points. For the two treatments below, each of which can be done in about ten minutes, you'll use either a tumbled gemstone, crystal, or wand to apply pressure to those points, promoting circulation while also helping to release toxins from the body and relaxing it.

What you'll need:

- ♦ Terry cloth towel
- ♦ Gem oil elixir
- ♦ Amethyst wand or tumbled stone with a smooth edge

CHAKRA ENERGY HAND MASSAGE

This treatment can be completed in less than ten minutes. However, if any of the chakra points feels tender, I advise you to work on it for longer, since this is typically a sign that the point needs extra attention.

Corresponding chakras for hand points:

1 Root chakra

2 Sacral chakra

3 Solar Plexus chakra

4 Heart chakra

5 Throat chakra

6 Third Eye chakra

7 Crown chakra

1. Gently apply a charged oil elixir to your hand and forearm and towel off any excess oil from your hands.

2. Starting with the right hand, using the broad end of a gemstone wand, slowly glide the wand up from the wrist toward the elbow and shoulder. Apply moderate to light pressure on the upward stroke, and lighten the pressure when gliding over your joints and bones. When you reach your shoulder, release pressure on the wand but remain in contact with the skin as you glide it back to the beginning point of the stroke. Repeat three times.

3. Use the broad end of the gemstone wand to gently stimulate each of the seven chakra points. Begin with the Root chakra. Slowly ease pressure into the point and hold for 5 to 10 seconds (or as long as comfortable).

4. Slowly release pressure, glide to the next chakra point, and repeat on each successive point.

5. Holding the gemstone wand horizontally, glide over the palm of the hand three times. Repeat on the left arm and hand.

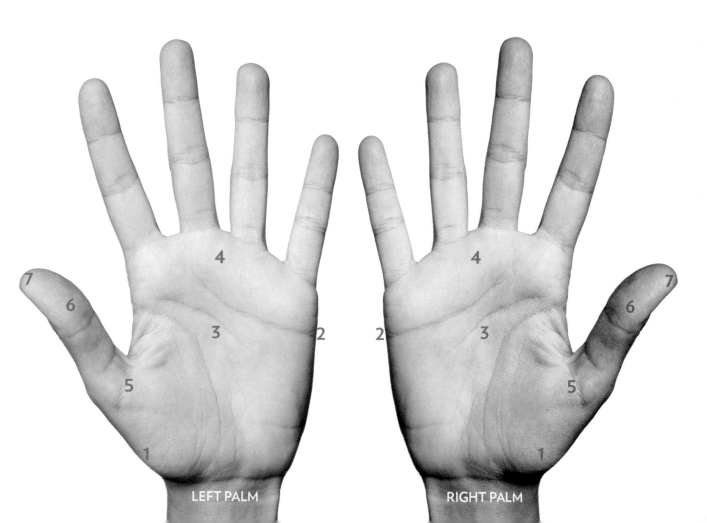

LEFT PALM   RIGHT PALM

CHAKRA FOOT MASSAGE

This massage helps to open energy channels in the feet, stimulating the chakras and organs.

Corresponding chakras for foot points:

1 Root chakra

2 Sacral chakra

3 Solar Plexus chakra

4 Heart chakra

5 Throat chakra

6 Third Eye chakra

7 Crown chakra

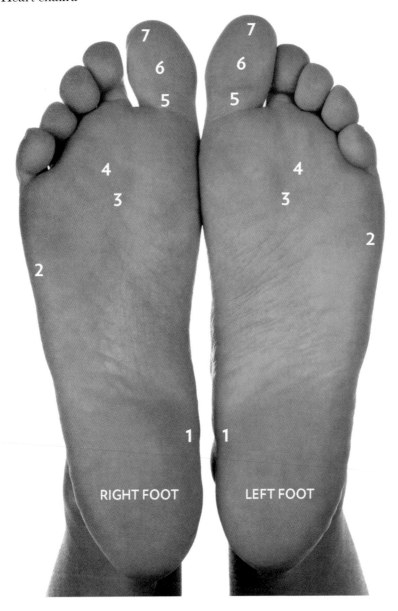

RIGHT FOOT   LEFT FOOT

1. Gently apply a charged oil elixir to the tops and soles of your feet up to the knee and towel off any excess oil.

2. Starting with the right foot, using the broad end of a gemstone wand, slowly glide the wand up from the ankle to just below the knee. Apply moderate to light pressure on the upward stroke, and lighten the pressure when gliding over your joints and bones. When you reach below the knee, release pressure on the wand but remain in contact with the skin as you glide it back to the beginning point of the stroke. Repeat three times.

3. Use the broad end of the gemstone wand to gently stimulate each of the seven chakra points. Begin with the Root chakra. Slowly ease pressure into the point and hold for 5 to 10 seconds (or as long as comfortable).

4. Slowly release pressure, glide to the next point, and repeat on each successive point.

5. Holding the gemstone wand horizontally, glide over the sole of the foot three times. Repeat on the left foot.

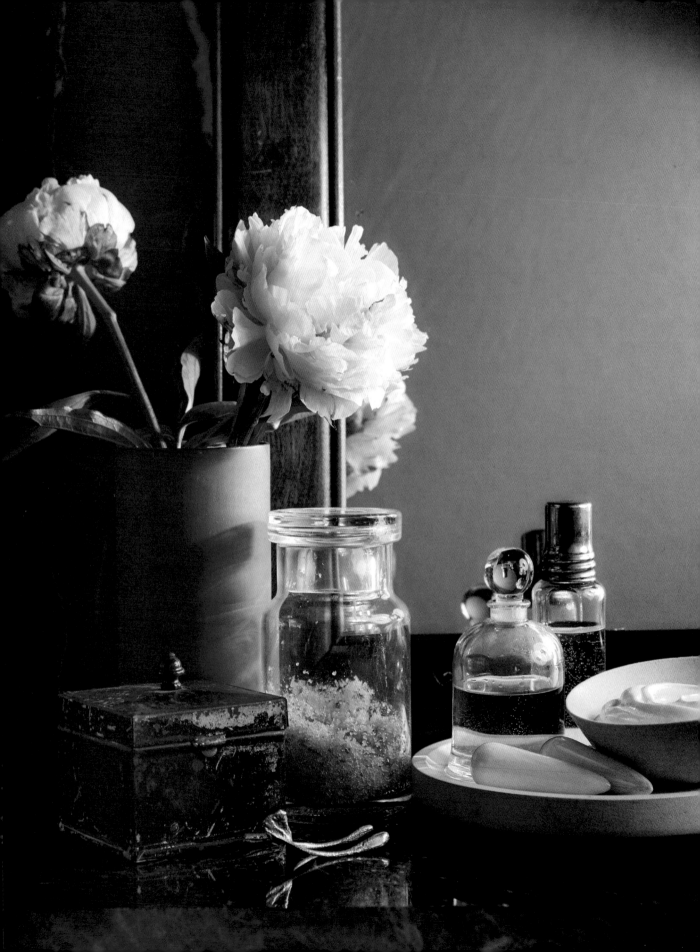

REBALANCE, RESTORE, RECHARGE

GEMSTONE FACE AND BODY TREATMENTS

Of all the chapters in this book, this is the one I'm most excited to share with you. I've spent the past fifteen years experimenting with gemstones and crystals as well as precious metals in various face and body treatments, and I've seen firsthand the transformative effects they have on all types of skin. People tell me my skin looks great for someone in her forties, which is nice to hear, of course. Trust me, though, there are still many days I wake up after having eaten a bag of chips or having stayed awake most of the night thinking about a big meeting the following day and look in the mirror and think, *Where did those dark under-eye circles come from?* or *Why does my skin look so dull?* For me, the goal is not "perfect skin," because I don't believe in such a thing, but healthy skin. I want to be able to effectively treat and soothe imperfections so that I put my best face forward every day. As our lifestyle and habits vary, so does our skin, which is why I don't believe there's any such thing as "bad skin" as much as I believe in balancing and restoring our skin.

My mother has always been my skincare role model because of her dedicated routine and no-sun policy—and that routine has paid off. She's now in her seventies, but you'd never know it from looking at her. Before I went off to college, she and I had a wonderful bonding ritual: after I finished my homework or on weekends, we would raid the kitchen pantry and refrigerator to create DIY concoctions—from face and hair masks to exfoliants. No matter how often we did it, I was always amazed at the magic that would result from using simple ingredients like oatmeal, olive oil, honey, sugar, and other grocery staples to smooth, hydrate, and brighten our skin or condition our hair. Of course, both my mother and I have learned a tremendous amount about ingredients since then, and we've built our brand by combining ancient healing traditions that utilize crystals, gemstones, and precious metals with the biotechnology to help restore, revitalize, and nourish the skin while also feeding the senses and the soul.

Like the ingredients in the concoctions I once whipped up in my kitchen with my mom, those in the recipes that follow serve a specific purpose. For example, gold and silver colloidals have natural antimicrobial and antibacterial properties that help to harmonize and balance the skin. The gemstone and crystal elixirs help to brighten and clarify. They also allow you to experience subtle gemstone energy infused with the intention of the programmed elixir. This is why it's always so important to give thought to your intention— whether it's protection, love, or spiritual harmony—before programming or charging your elixir. You can even write the intention down on a sticky note or label and tape it to the storage bottle or jar to help further enhance and remind (think Dr. Emoto).

All of the ingredients in the recipes that follow can be purchased online, and many are also available at health food stores or grocery stores (see the resource guide on page 215 for retailers). I recommend buying organic products whenever possible, as it's always better to use ingredients free and clear of chemicals and pesticides. If your skin is sensitive, it's a good idea to test a recipe first by applying a quarter-size dab of the cleanser, mask, or tonic directly below the jawline to see how your skin might react. All of these recipes can be adapted to meet your needs.

I hope by now I've convinced you that spending a little extra time on skincare is well worth the effort. I invite you to take some time alone or with a friend to prepare these recipes and allow them to work their magic on your skin. In doing such, you'll clear your mind while nourishing your spirit, so you'll feel as revitalized as your skin looks.

GEMSTONE CLEANSERS, TONICS, MASKS, AND SCRUBS

PEARL RICE CLEANSING POWDER

This cleansing powder can be used day or night as part of your skincare routine. Rice powders and cleansing oils have been used for centuries, and they continue to gain new devotees today because they're equal parts gentle and effective. This recipe combines the best of both a powder and an oil cleanser. Vitamin C and pearl powders illuminate and soften the skin. Depending on how hydrated or dry your skin is on any given day, you can change up the treatment to achieve optimal results. Bear in mind that this can be affected by a number of factors including hormones, sleep, nutrition, stress level, climate, and travel. Hydrated skin looks and feels glowing, luminous, and balanced, while dry or dehydrated skin lacks tone and has more prominent fine lines and wrinkles. If skin is fatigued, you may notice dark under-eye circles, breakouts, blotchiness, or dryness.

Skin type: Customizable for all types; use daily

Purpose: Gently exfoliates, cleanses, and tones without stripping the skin of natural oils or leaving a residue

For the powder cleanser:

- 1 teaspoon rice powder (or rice flour)
- ⅛ teaspoon vitamin C powder (for more sensitive skin, use just a pinch or omit)
- ¼ teaspoon pearl powder

In a small glass or ceramic bowl, combine the rice powder, vitamin C powder, and pearl powder.

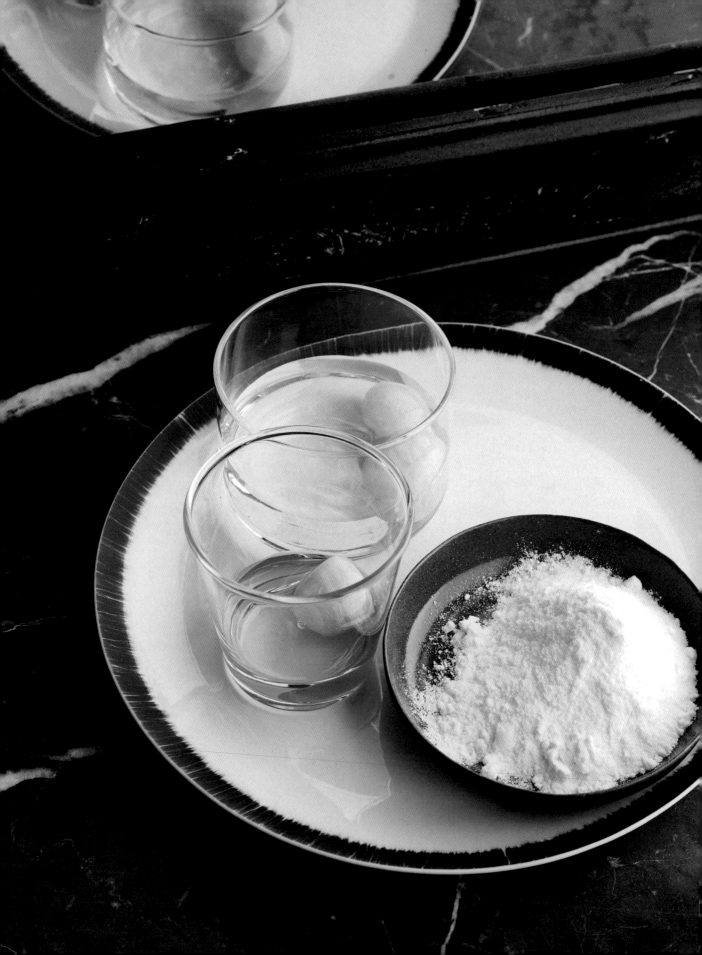

For the liquid cleanser:

- ♦ ¼ teaspoon rose quartz water elixir (see chapter 4)

- ♦ 1–2 drops rose quartz oil elixir (optional, for normal to dry skin)

- ♦ ½ teaspoon pure organic aloe vera gel (optional, for oily or combination skin)

Wet your face with warm water and then dry your hands. Add the rose quartz water elixir (including the rose quartz oil elixir and/or aloe vera gel, as desired) to the powder mixture. Apply the cleansing powder to your face, avoiding the eye area. Gently exfoliate damp skin by moving your fingertips in a circular motion wherever the powder is for 30 to 60 seconds. Rinse off the powder with luke warm water.

GEMSTONE-IN-THE-ROUND

Pearls have symbolized wealth and status for thousands of years. A Chinese historian recorded the oldest written mention of natural pearls in 2206 BCE. From those ancient times until Christopher Columbus's voyages in 1492, pearls could be found in the Persian Gulf, the waters of Ceylon (now Sri Lanka), Chinese rivers and lakes, and the rivers of Europe. Columbus himself discovered natural pearl sources in the waters of present-day Venezuela and Panama.

Still considered treasures from the earth's ponds, lakes, seas, and oceans, pearls have a natural resonancy with lunar and tidal forces that continues to embody the mystery, power, and life-sustaining nature of water.

Pearls are natural antioxidants containing amino acids, minerals, and proteins that help to purify, replenish, and rebuild the skin's natural collagen. Ground pearl powder has been used in facial treatments dating back to ancient Egypt, China, and Japan to help brighten, even, and perfect the skin.

CALMING AMETHYST TONIC

If your skin is at all irritated or inflamed, this may very well become your go-to tonic. Amethyst, aloe, and silver are known for their natural cooling and antibacterial properties. Silver is still used in hospitals today for wound healing. Lavender helps calm skin while also alleviating irritation. Not only is this tonic great for soothing sensitized skin, but also you can use a few spritzes of the tonic to set makeup or as an afternoon pick-me-up.

Skin type: Normal, oily, combination, or irritated; use daily or as often as desired

Purpose: Balances, refreshes, and calms skin

- ½ cup amethyst water elixir
- ¼ teaspoon silver colloidal
- ½ tablespoon pure organic aloe vera gel or juice
- Pinch of Himalayan salt (preferred) or sea salt
- 1–3 drops lavender or chamomile essential oil

In a small glass or ceramic bowl, combine the amethyst water elixir with the silver colloidal, aloe vera gel or juice, and salt. Then add the essential oil. Place the mixture in an atomizer (preferred) or a glass bottle.

Use this tonic after cleansing. If you have an atomizer, gently mist the tonic onto your skin. Alternatively, gently press the tonic onto the skin with your fingertips in gentle fluttering motions.

Pure Aloe Vera Gel
I'm sure many of us have a plastic bottle of bright green "aloe vera gel" hanging out somewhere in one of our bathroom or medicine cabinets, bought in haste at the drugstore after a beach day gone awry. You know the stuff. Unfortunately, that "aloe vera gel" is mostly alcohol—mixed with a whole host of other nasty chemicals. Not only will it do little to truly soothe sunburn (it may even exacerbate it by drying out the skin), it is especially terrible for the delicate skin on your face, throat, and décolletage. When I call for pure organic aloe vera gel here, I'm talking about undiluted aloe vera gel, which you can find at health food stores and many markets. Just check the ingredients list on the side of the bottle. You're looking for 100 percent organic aloe vera—nothing else. Once you open a bottle of pure aloe vera gel, store it in the refrigerator both for longevity and for added cooling upon application.

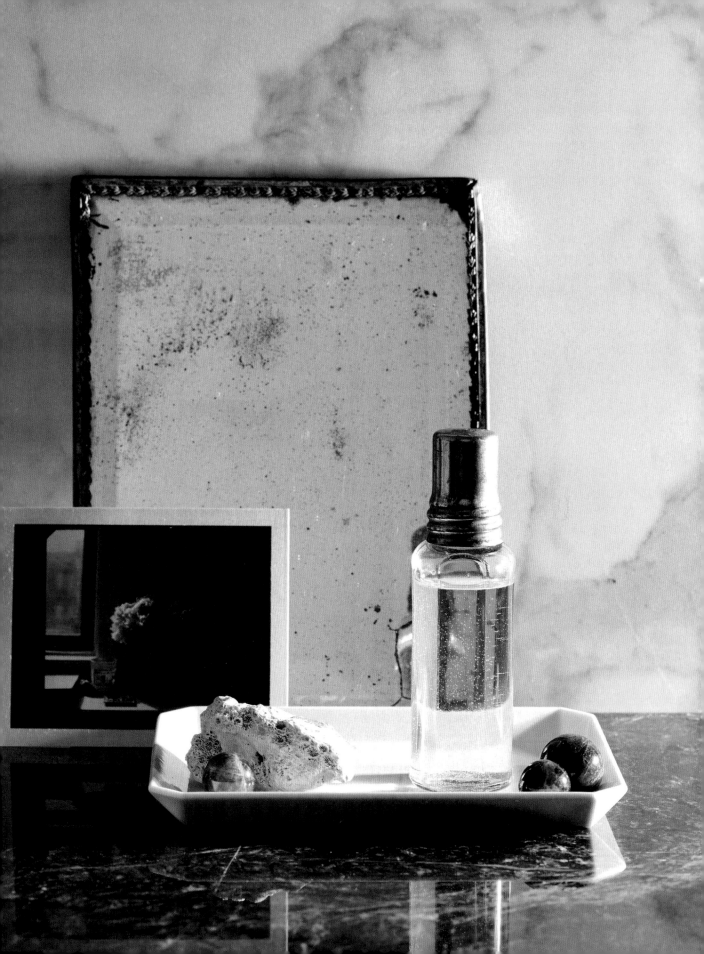

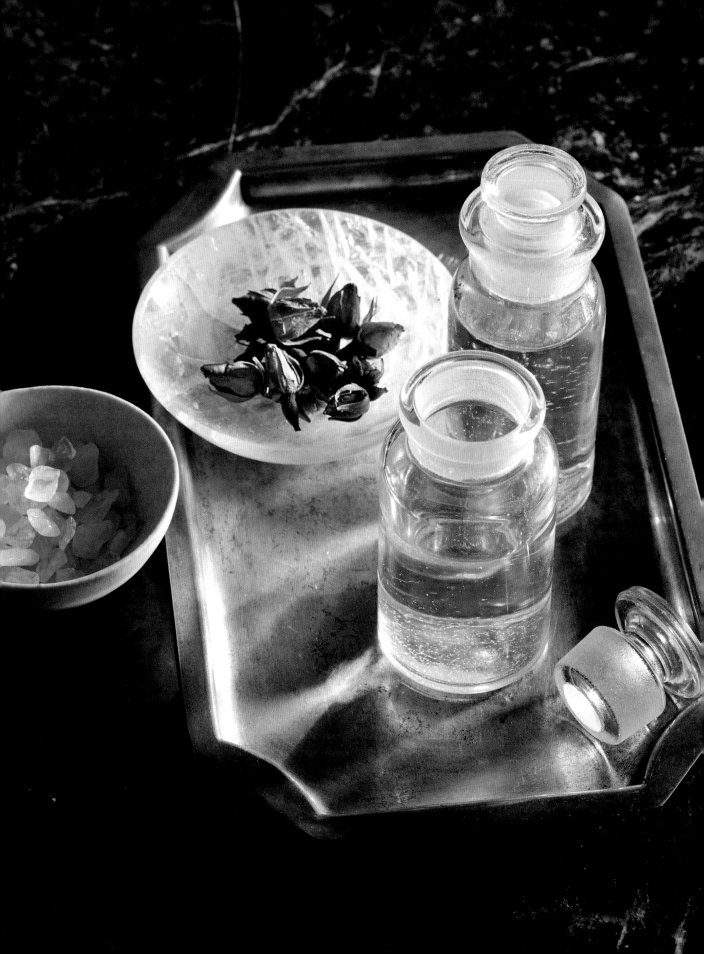

ROSE GOLD TONIC

This tonic works wonders on dull, dry skin, so mix up a batch after a long flight or on days you spend too much time indoors. Both rose and gold have been used to treat skin since ancient times, and with good reason. Rose hydrates and soothes, while gold colloidal is known for its regenerative and energizing properties. During the summer months, you can store the tonic in the refrigerator and use it as a cooling, energizing body mist.

Skin type: Dry and/or sensitive; use daily or as needed

Purpose: Leaves the skin feeling soft and protected

- ½ cup rose quartz water elixir
- ¼ teaspoon gold colloidal
- ½ tablespoon pure organic aloe vera gel or juice
- Pinch of Himalayan salt (preferred) or sea salt
- 1–3 drops rose, geranium, and/or ylang-ylang essential oil

In a small glass or ceramic bowl, combine the rose quartz water elixir with the gold colloidal, aloe vera gel or juice, and salt. Then add the essential oil. Place the mixture in an atomizer (preferred) or glass bottle.

Use this tonic after cleansing. If you have an atomizer, gently mist the tonic onto your skin. Alternatively, press the tonic onto the skin with your fingertips in gentle fluttering motions.

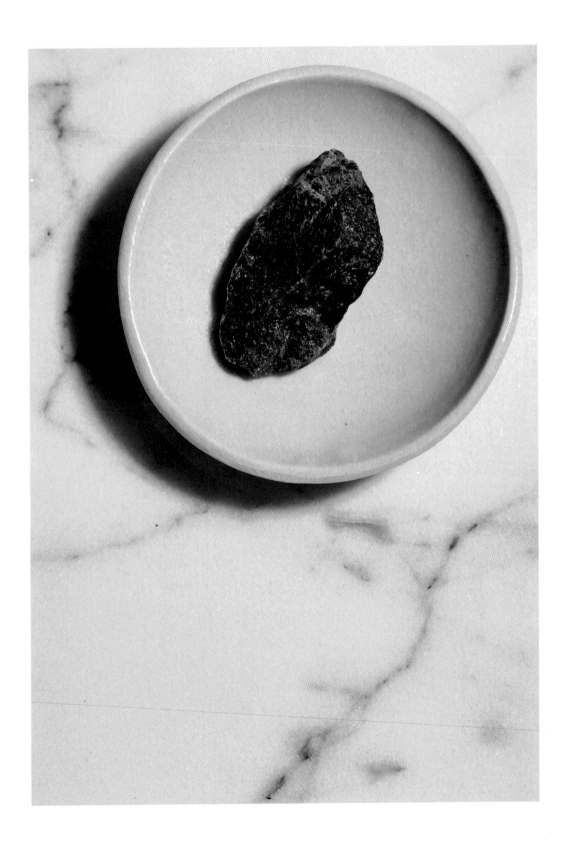

SKIN REVITALIZERS: PRECIOUS METALS

You wear jewelry made with gold, silver, and copper, but it may never have occurred to you to use them in your skincare. Gold, silver, and copper all have long medicinal and healing histories. Over the years, I've discovered how potent these precious metals are. Gold is known to regenerate aging or damaged skin cells, while silver nurtures and copper renews and energizes dull, tired skin. An effective way to incorporate precious metals into your skincare routine is to purchase them in colloidal form.

GOLD

Universally cherished, gold was held in high esteem by many cultures as early as the fourth millennium BCE. The earliest therapeutic application of gold can be traced back to 2500 BCE in China where gold was used to treat smallpox, skin ulcers, and measles. Japanese tradition suggests that thin gold foils placed into tea, sake, and food may be beneficial to your health. Since the 1920s, gold and gold complexes have been used to treat a wide range of ailments, from pulmonary tuberculosis to rheumatoid arthritis.

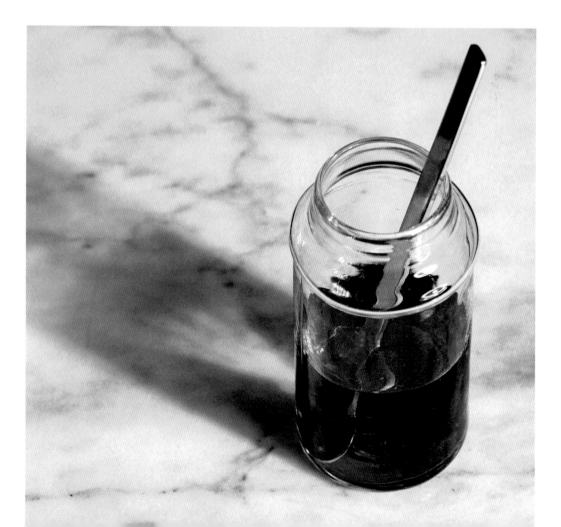

More recently, gold complexes have been explored for effectiveness against acute forms of asthma, arthritis, and nerve-related illnesses. Current research has also described promising results in using gold complexes to treat cancer. Gold has become a go-to ingredient in skincare products because of its antiaging and regenerative properties. In fact, gold acts like a small charger, because it's metal and we have electricity in our bodies. As such, it's good for restoring the lost elasticity of the body's tissue.

SILVER

This precious metal was first mined in about 3000 BCE in Anatolia (modern-day Turkey). Its luster has long been thought to mirror the soul, enhancing intuitive energy. In ancient Greece, Hippocrates, the "father of medicine," knew of its healing and antidisease properties. It is said that he used silver on himself to treat ulcers and to expedite wound healing. Thousands of years later, during World War I, before the advent of antibiotics, silver was an important weapon against disease on the battlefield. More recently, silver is used in wound dressings and creams and as an antibiotic coating on medical devices. Silver's antimicrobial and antibacterial properties make it a prime candidate to treat skin ailments including acne.

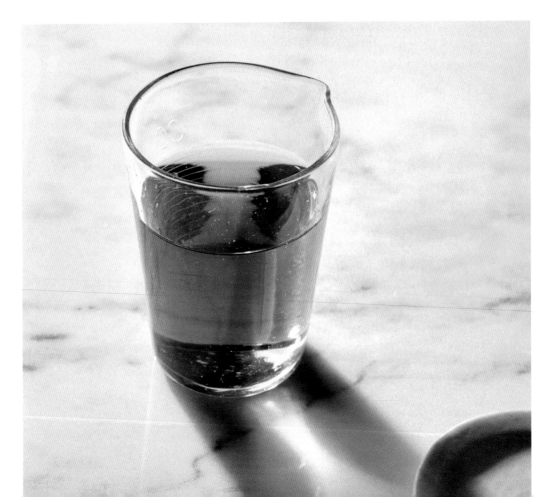

COPPER

Copper's history dates back more than ten thousand years. In legend, copper is said to be the metal of the god Hermes, who facilitates mental agility and quick wit. Copper was first used to sterilize wounds sometime between 2600 and 2200 BCE. Other early reports of copper's medicinal uses include using copper compounds for headaches, "trembling of the limbs" (perhaps referring to epilepsy), and burns. By the reign of Roman emperor Tiberius (14 to 37 CE), copper and its derivatives had been firmly established as an important drug. The first modern research on the subject of copper's medicinal use was done by Professor John R. J. Sorenson of the University of Arkansas for Medical Sciences, College of Pharmacy. In 1966, Dr. Sorenson demonstrated that copper complexes can be used to treat inflammatory diseases. Since then, copper complexes have been used to successfully treat patients with arthritic and other chronic degenerative diseases. When it comes to your skin, a copper deficiency can result in wrinkles, crow's-feet, varicose veins, and saggy skin. Certain peptides, the small fragments of proteins that serve as the key building blocks of most living tissues, have an affinity for copper, to which they bind very tightly. The resulting compound has become known as a copper peptide. When infused in skincare products, copper peptides are said to improve the elastic fiber in skin, increase skin flexibility, and act as an antiwrinkle treatment.

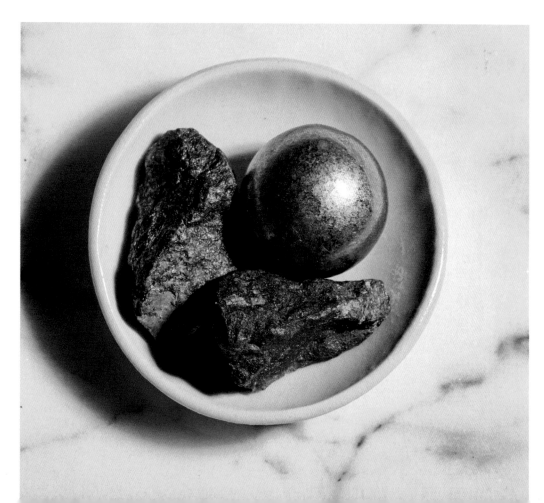

CHARCOAL AND SILVER DETOX MASK

This deep-cleaning mask acts like a magnet to extract impurities from the skin including environmental toxins, dirt, and debris. The activated charcoal attracts and binds to metals, chemicals, and toxins, while the colloidal silver and bentonite clay help kill bacteria. You can always use a foundation brush or fan brush to spread the mask over your face and neck, ensuring a thick, even application. But fingers work just fine, too!

Skin type: All, especially oily or combination skin; use once per week, or as needed

Purpose: Helps to detox and purify the skin

- ◆ 2 capsules of activated charcoal
- ◆ 1 teaspoon bentonite clay
- ◆ 1 teaspoon (heaping) pure organic aloe vera gel
- ◆ ⅛ teaspoon silver colloidal

Break open the charcoal capsules and empty their contents into a small glass or ceramic bowl. Add the bentonite clay, aloe vera gel, and silver colloidal to the charcoal, mixing with a wooden spoon.

On cleansed skin, gently smooth a thick layer of the mask over the neck and face, avoiding the eye area. Allow the mask to sit for 5 to 8 minutes. Rinse off the mask with warm water or remove it with a damp soft cloth. Gently pat your face dry.

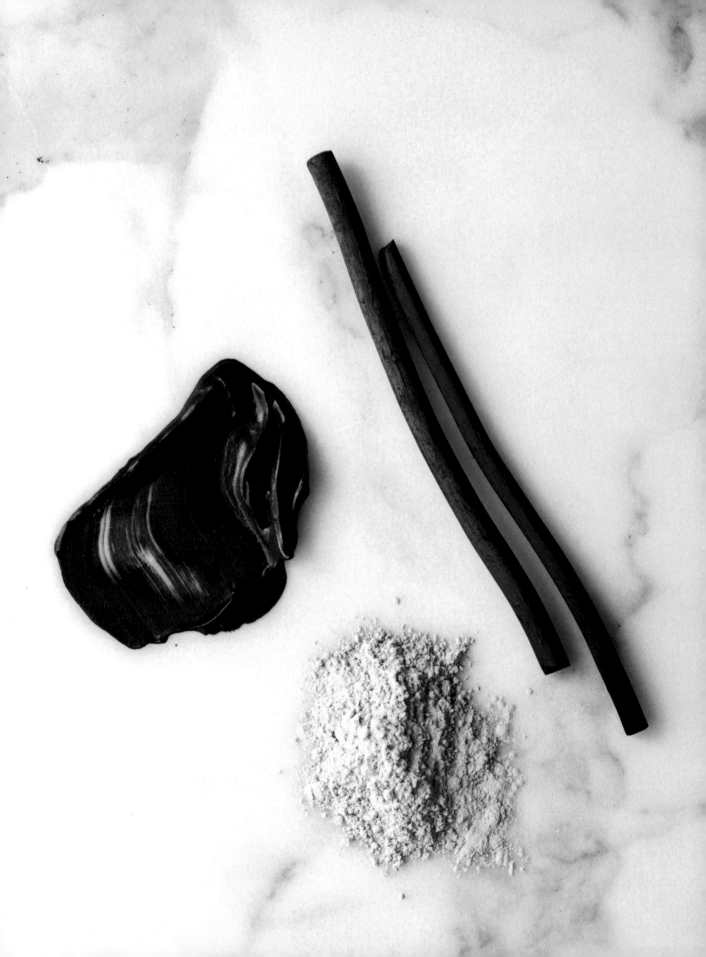

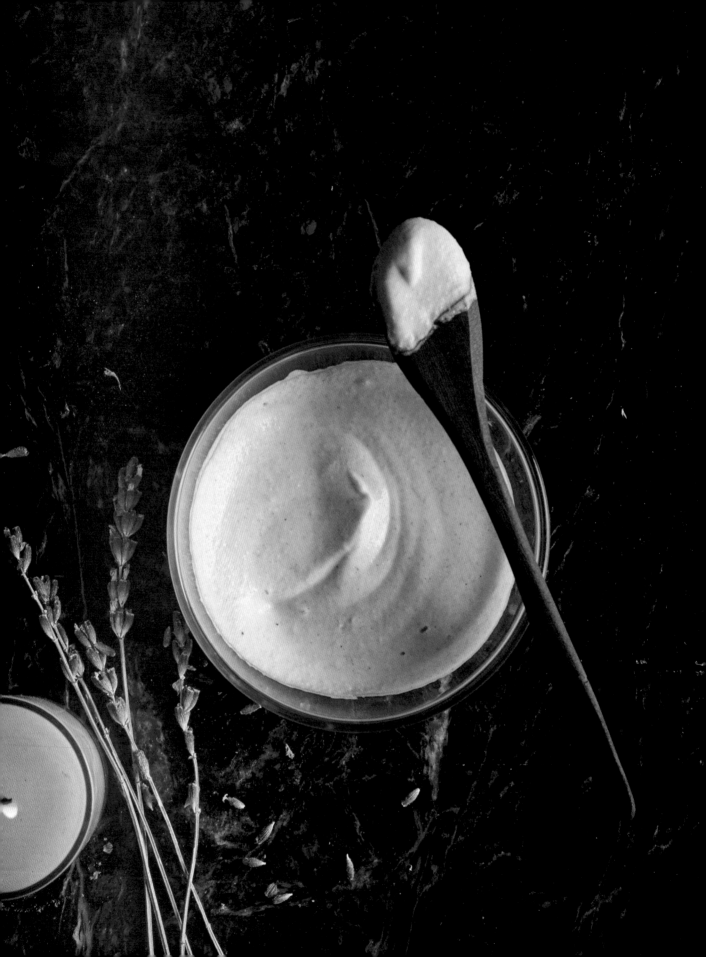

SOOTHING GEMSTONE AND OAT MASK

Whether you live in a dry climate or your skin is chapped from cold weather, this mask provides a deep level of calming and soothing. It combines naturally soothing ingredients such as oatmeal and silver colloidal with amethyst elixir, which is known for its rebalancing and harmonizing properties. For extra soothing and to help the mask penetrate the skin, use an atomizer to spray a few spritzes of tonic on your face before applying.

Skin type: All; use one or two times per week

Purpose: Brings relief and balance to irritated skin

- 1½ tablespoons ground organic oatmeal
- 1 tablespoon amethyst, blue lace agate, or aquamarine water elixir
- 1 tablespoon pure organic aloe vera gel
- 1 tablespoon plain Greek yogurt
- ¼ teaspoon silver colloidal
- 1 drop lavender or chamomile essential oil

In a small glass or ceramic bowl, combine the oatmeal, gem water elixir, aloe vera gel, Greek yogurt, silver colloidal, and essential oil, mixing with a wooden spoon.

On cleansed skin, gently smooth a thick layer of the mask over the neck and face, avoiding the eye area. Allow the mask to sit for 5 to 10 minutes. Rinse off the mask with warm water or remove it with a damp soft cloth. Gently pat your face dry.

ILLUMINATING MASK

After a day when you eat poorly or a night when you don't get enough sleep, your skin often pays the price, appearing dull and ashy. This mask will bring it back to life and make you look glowing and well rested, thanks to ingredients such as pearl and lemon, which brighten the skin's appearance while also helping to detoxify. For extra skin softening, you can leave the mask on for a few minutes longer, allowing the lactic acid from the yogurt to gently exfoliate your skin.

Skin type: All; use once per week, or as needed

Purpose: Brightens and evens skin tone

- 1 tablespoon plain Greek yogurt
- ¼ teaspoon freshly squeezed lemon juice
- ¼ teaspoon pearl powder
- ⅛ teaspoon gold colloidal
- ½ teaspoon pure organic aloe vera gel
- Pinch of vitamin C powder (optional)

In a small glass or ceramic bowl, combine the yogurt, lemon juice, pearl powder, gold colloidal, aloe vera gel, and vitamin C powder (if using), mixing with a wooden spoon.

On cleansed skin, gently smooth a thick layer of the mask over the neck and face, avoiding the eye area. Allow the mask to sit for 5 to 8 minutes. Rinse off the mask with warm water or remove it with a damp soft cloth. Gently pat your face dry.

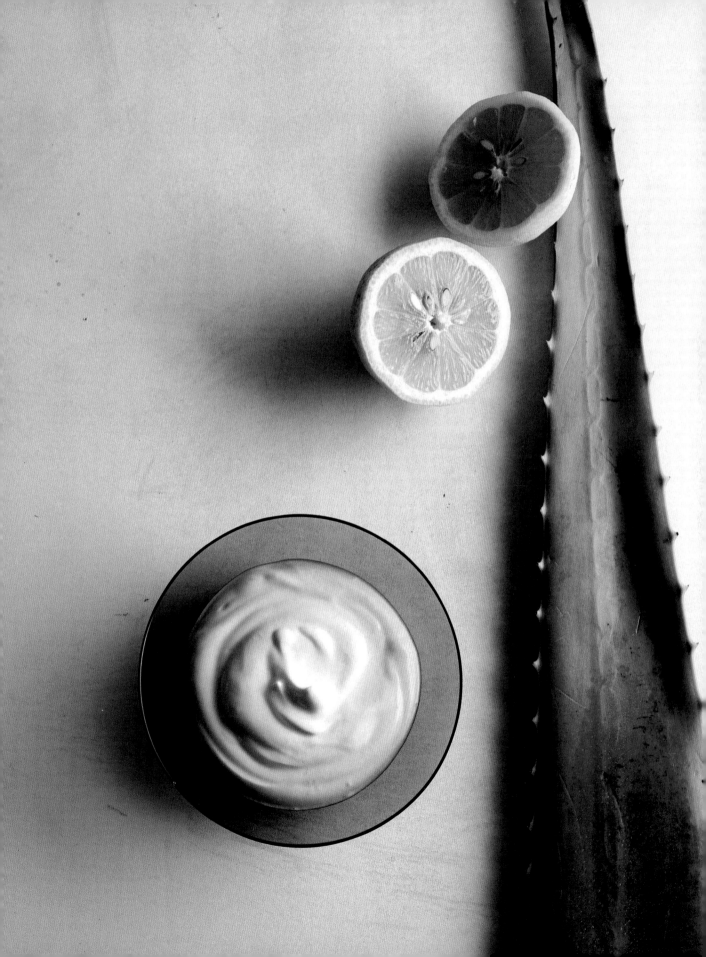

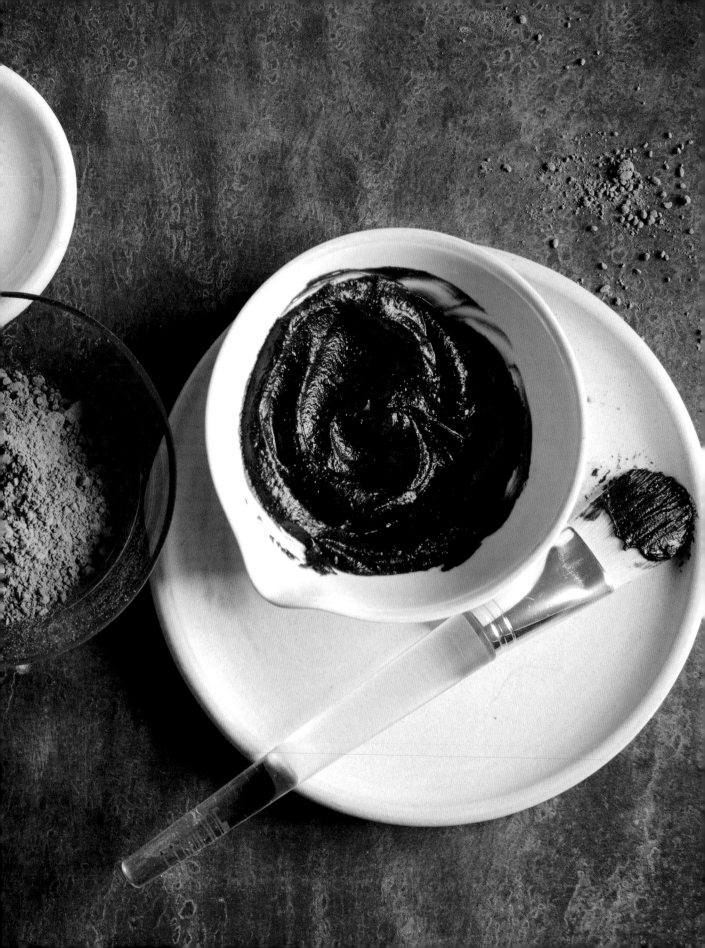

GOLD MATCHA FIRMING MASK

This treatment is ideal for aging skin, since it combines the regenerative aspects of gold with the antioxidant power of matcha (powdered green tea), which keep skin plumped and hydrated while fighting against the negative effects of UV radiation. Honey is also a key player. In addition to its antifungal, antiviral, and anti-inflammatory properties, the sweet nectar also contains gluconic acid, which is known to brighten dull skin. Consider having a cup of matcha while the mask is on your face—the polyphenols it contains have been tied to protection against heart disease and cancer as well as blood pressure reduction and antiaging.

Skin type: All; use once per week, or as needed

Purpose: Tones, firms, and leaves skin glowing

- ½ teaspoon matcha
- ½ teaspoon gold colloidal
- ⅛ teaspoon copper colloidal (optional)
- ½ teaspoon raw organic honey or organic honey

In a small glass or ceramic bowl, combine the matcha, colloidal(s), and honey, mixing with a wooden spoon.

On cleansed skin, gently smooth a thick layer of the mask over the neck and face, avoiding the eye area. Allow it to sit for 10 to 15 minutes. Rinse off the mask with warm water or remove it with a damp soft cloth. Gently pat your face dry.

Matcha

Matcha is a powder made entirely of ground green tea leaves. With typical green tea preparation, you steep the tea leaves in hot water, infusing the water and then discarding the leaves. But with matcha, you are consuming—or applying, as the case may be—the entire tea leaf and therefore ingesting or absorbing far more of its powerful antioxidant properties. Just be careful to look for pure matcha powder. Because matcha has a strong, grassy taste that some people find too strong, it often comes premixed with sugar or other sweeteners.

SPIRULINA ANTIAGING MASK

Whether you're looking to prevent the signs of aging (wrinkles, fine lines, etc.) or to treat existing ones, this mask is the one to turn to. It contains spirulina, a type of blue-green algae rich in protein, vitamins, minerals, carotenoids, and antioxidants that can help protect cells from damage, along with reparative aloe to replace lost moisture. For extra-dry skin, apply a thin veil of oil elixir—or a light carrier oil—on your skin before applying the mask.

Skin type: All; use once per week, or more as needed

Purpose: Promotes radiant, smooth, and youthful skin

- 1 teaspoon organic spirulina powder
- 1 tablespoon pure organic aloe vera gel
- ¼ teaspoon gold colloidal
- ½ teaspoon amethyst or clear or rose quartz water elixir

In a small glass or ceramic bowl, combine the spirulina powder, aloe vera gel, gold colloidal, and gem water elixir, mixing with a wooden spoon.

On cleansed skin, gently smooth a thick layer of the mask all over the neck and face, avoiding the eye area. Allow it to sit for 10 to 15 minutes. Rinse off the mask with warm water or remove it with a damp soft cloth. Gently pat your face dry.

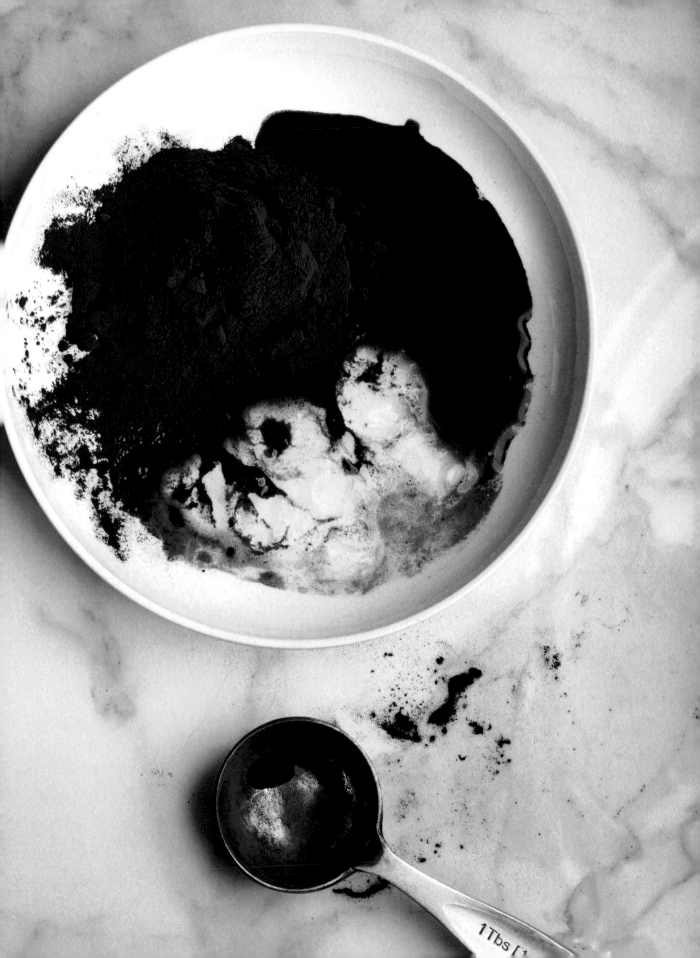

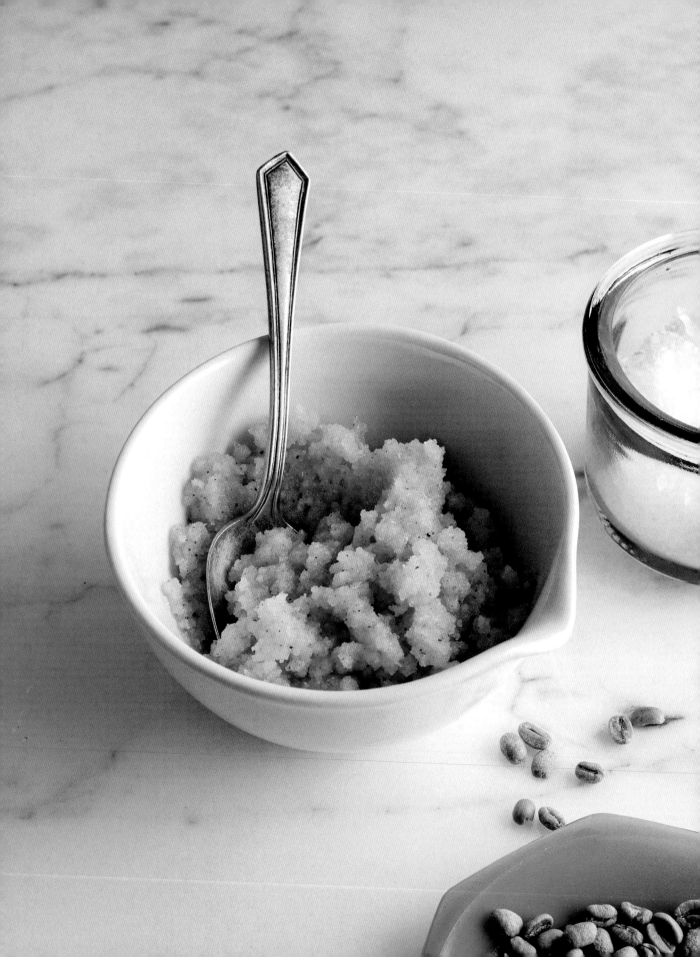

COCO GOLD BODY SCRUB

Caffeine not only helps us perk up in the morning, but it also can combat signs of skin fatigue by increasing microcirculation in skin cells. The result is more firmness and elasticity. This luxurious body scrub combines the toning and energizing benefits of green coffee with rich coconut oil, gold colloidal, and sea salt for the perfect polish. If you prefer an unscented scrub, you can swap out the coconut oil for avocado oil.

Skin type: All; use daily, or as needed

Purpose: Softens, hydrates, and invigorates skin

- 3–4 capsules of green coffee
- 1 cup sea salt
- ⅓ cup coconut oil elixir charged with your stone of choice
- ½ teaspoon gold colloidal

Break open the green coffee capsules and empty the contents into a medium glass or ceramic bowl. Add the sea salt, coconut oil elixir, and gold colloidal to the green coffee, mixing well with a wooden spoon. Scrape the scrub into a glass jar that has a resealable lid.

In the shower, apply a generous amount of the scrub all over the body (you can also use it on the face, but avoid the eye area). Rub gently in a clockwise circular motion to exfoliate dead skin cells. Rinse off the scrub with warm water or remove it with a damp soft cloth. Gently pat your skin dry.

HIMALAYAN ROSE BODY SCRUB

This body scrub combines the softening power of rose with the majestic and healing properties of Himalayan pink salt, rose quartz, and gold. To help clear the mind and body, try using a clear quartz oil elixir or blue sapphire oil elixir instead of rose quartz, and frankincense essential oil instead of a flower essential oil.

Skin type: All; use daily, or as needed

Purpose: Calms skin while awakening the spirit

- 1 cup Himalayan pink salt
- ⅓ cup rose quartz oil elixir
- ½ teaspoon gold colloidal
- 3 tablespoons crushed dried rose buds
- 5–10 drops flower essential oil such as rose, ylang-ylang, or chamomile

In a small glass or ceramic bowl, combine the salt, oil elixir, gold colloidal, dried rose buds, and essential oil, mixing well with a wooden spoon.

Apply a generous amount of the scrub to the skin either just before showering or once in the shower. Rub gently in circular motions to exfoliate dead skin cells. Rinse off the scrub with warm water or remove it with a damp soft cloth. Gently pat your skin dry.

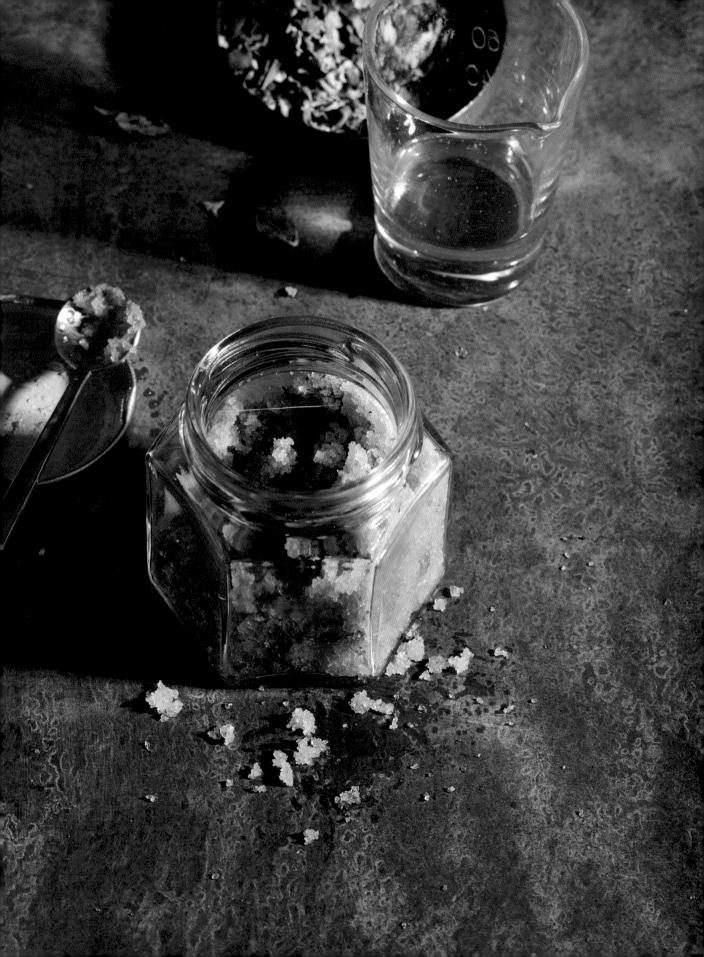

GEMSTONE STEAMS

You may have tried DIY steams that involve placing your towel-draped head directly over a pot filled with recently boiled water (using the towel to trap the steam). But you've likely never infused your steam with gemstone and crystal energy. Gemstone facial steams revitalize the skin while also heightening the senses. The steams are also an easy way to boost circulation and bring oxygen to the skin while softening and loosening any debris. They are perfect for preparing your skin for masks or other treatments. The suggested gemstone and crystal facial steams below pair various stones with essential oils, herbs, and/or flowers. Use any of the suggested combinations, then follow the general steam instructions for safely creating the ideal gemstone facial steam for your skin's needs.

TIP: As a rule of thumb, use 3 to 4 drops of essential oil and a handful of dried herbs or flowers for steams. If you prefer a stronger scent, use 4 to 6 drops of oil.

HEALING AND REBALANCING

- Purple stones
- Dried lavender and/or lavender essential oil
- ½ teaspoon silver colloidal (optional)

CALMING

- Blue stones
- Dried chamomile and/or chamomile essential oil

DECONGESTING

- Green moss agate
- Dried eucalyptus or rosemary and/or eucalyptus or rosemary essential oil

SOOTHING AND HYDRATING

- Rose quartz
- Dried rose buds and/or rose or ylang-ylang essential oil
- ½ teaspoon gold colloidal (optional)

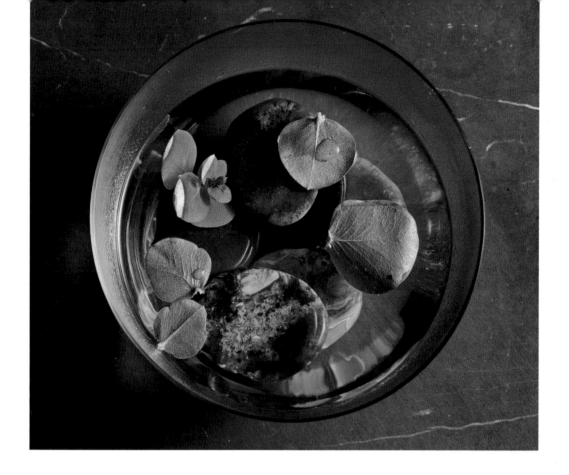

HOW TO DO A GEMSTONE FACIAL STEAM

1. Using a pot with a ceramic-lined interior, fill it with approximately 4 to 5 cups of water. Carefully submerge your gemstones of choice. Heat the pot on medium-high until the water reaches a slow boil, then immediately remove the pot from the heat.

2. Carefully transfer the boiling water and stones from your pot into a large glass or ceramic bowl. Add a handful of herbs or flowers of your choosing and 3 to 4 drops of essential oil (or more, according to your personal preference). Add the colloidals if using them. Allow the ingredients to steep.

3. Once the water cools to approximately 110 to 116°F (give it around 5 minutes), place your face about 6 to 8 inches from the surface of the water (or at a distance that feels comfortable; the steam should feel soothing—not too hot). Loosely place a towel over your head and around the bowl, creating a tent so that the steam does not escape.

4. Gently steam your skin for 5 to 10 minutes (no more than 5 minutes if your skin is particularly sensitive or easily aggravated).

5. Gently splash your face with lukewarm water. At this point you can apply a mask or a hydrating product, or simply pat your skin dry with a soft towel.

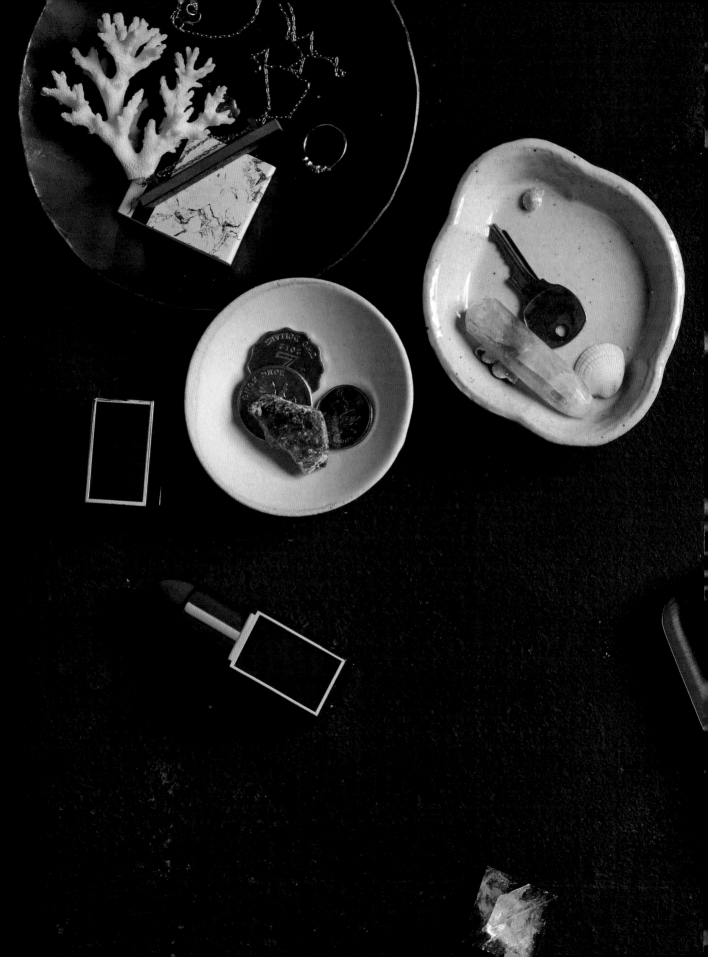

9

PERFECT RESONANCE

FINDING GEMSTONES FOR YOUR LIFESTYLE

I've amassed hundreds of stones over the years, both for business and pleasure, and I can honestly say there are only a handful—five or maybe six—with which I truly resonate. So if you haven't felt a strong connection with any stone just yet, I encourage you to give it more time. While a crystal's or gem's energy remains consistent, yours does not; if you're not "clicking" with a particular stone on a specific day, try again on another. It may also be possible that you haven't found *your* stone yet. Give it time and keep an open mind—the energy within gemstones and crystals often allows them to find you depending on your specific needs.

How will you know when you have found your ideal mineral match, or matches? The particular crystal or gemstone may send a gentle energetic tingle up your arm when you hold it in the palm of your hand. It may make you feel calm and grounded, sharp and clear-minded, or simply ready to take on the world. I like to call on those calming, clarifying powers wherever I am by wearing my favorite gemstones and crystals or placing them around my home, workplace, or home-away-from-home when I travel. Doing so improves the environment while also harmonizing the energy flow.

There are so many ways to wear crystals and gemstones for beauty *and* power, and even more ways to decorate with them for a lovely *and* healing home. What follows in this chapter are my suggestions for finding the perfect stones to wear or display, whatever your personal style and decor.

STONES TO WEAR

I have heard the expression at least a thousand times—you don't choose gemstone and crystal jewelry; it chooses you. And that may well be true, since we tend to gravitate toward what attracts us on a physical, emotional, or spiritual level. The first stone that ever chose you is your birthstone. But how authentic is that connection? After all, you're far from the only one born during a particular month. And just how did certain colors of stones become associated with the twelve months of the calendar year?

Many scholars believe that the origin of birthstones lies in the biblical story of Moses's brother, Aaron, who wore a breastplate embedded with twelve gemstones. The gems were said to represent the twelve tribes of Israel and to imbue the breastplate with a mystical protective power. The first-century Roman-Jewish historian Josephus was the first to link the stones of Aaron's breastplate to the zodiac, and later Christian scholars linked them to the twelve apostles. But our modern list of birthstones wasn't standardized until 1912, when the National Association of Jewelers published their definitive list—though in 1952 that list was updated by the Jewelry Industry Council of America. Still, you may notice that your birthstone varies, depending on which source you consult—and throughout history, accepted birthstones have rotated in and out, depending mainly on their availability and popularity.

> ### LITTLE GEM
>
> Wearing a crystal or gemstone ring on your dominant hand? Try turning it to face your palm on occasion. This will boost the powers of the energy pathways in that hand for healing and manifestation.

In the past, wearing a different birthstone other than the one designated to your birth month was believed to bring the wearer bad luck. However, just as the stones associated with certain months have changed over time, so have the superstitious beliefs that once surrounded them. Bottom line: If you gravitate toward a stone that isn't your birthstone, embrace it, or if you're at all superstitious, create a piece of custom jewelry with both your birthstone and another stone of your choice. Just keep in mind that a piece of jewelry that includes several different stones may cause conflict if the stones have widely differing effects (e.g., calming vs. energizing, or warming vs. cooling). Try to find—or design your own—pieces with stones that have similar properties or synergies. Likewise, wear opposing stones separately and at different times.

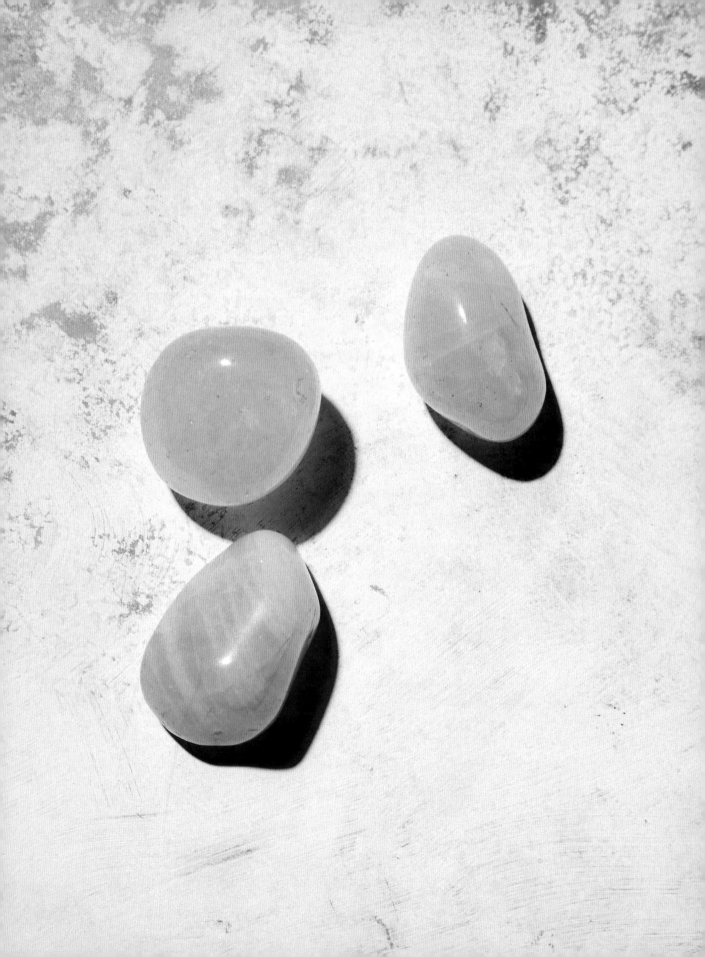

BIRTHSTONES

Here is the current list of birthstones and what they are said to bring to the wearer:

JANUARY	**Garnet:** Love, passion, sensuality, and intimacy
FEBRUARY	**Amethyst:** Peace, balance, courage, and inner strength
MARCH	**Aquamarine:** Release of fear, calming of nerves, and mental clarity
APRIL	**Diamond:** Purity, perfection, and authority
MAY	**Emerald:** Fidelity, enhanced memory, and intelligence
JUNE	**Pearl:** Purity, charity, integrity, truth, and loyalty **Moonstone (alternate):** Feminine energies, sensitivity, and intuition
JULY	**Ruby:** Integrity, devotion, and happiness
AUGUST	**Peridot:** Longevity, strong relationships, and mitigation of anger and jealousy
SEPTEMBER	**Sapphire:** Pain relief and personal expression
OCTOBER	**Pink tourmaline:** Flexibility, happiness, objectivity, compassion, serenity, and tolerance **Opal (alternate):** Love, hope, innocence, luck, and happiness
NOVEMBER	**Topaz:** Emotional balance and protection from greed **Citrine (alternate):** Success, clarity of thought, and abundance
DECEMBER	**Turquoise:** Healing and balancing **Tanzanite (alternate):** Spiritual awareness and psychic insight **Blue topaz (alternate):** Openness, honesty, self-realization, and self-control

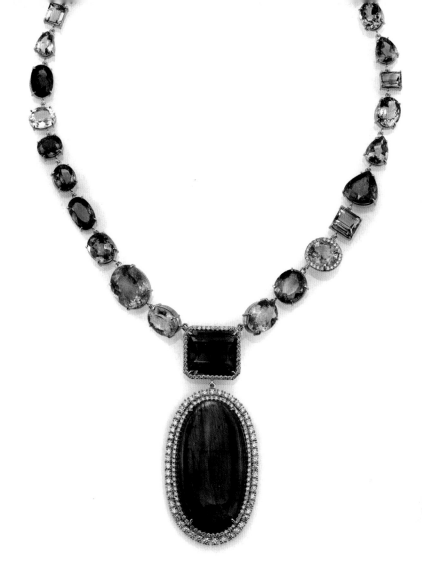

Whether you're drawn to your birthstone or another gemstone or crystal, committing to a fabulous piece of crystal or gemstone jewelry is an exciting prospect. And whether you want to have the emerald that was handed down from your great-grandmother made into a pendant, you're buying yourself a diamond ring rather than waiting for the perfect prospect to come along, or you simply love clarifying quartz jewelry, you can choose a setting that truly represents your personality and that you'll want to wear 24/7.

When it comes to *healing* jewelry, however, I've found that where you wear your stone matters. For instance, necklaces with shorter chains (14 to 18 inches in length) that lie closer to the throat can help to strengthen your personal voice, while necklaces with longer chains (22 to 30 inches) can actually impact matters of the heart. Whether buying a necklace or a ring, the setting you choose also plays a role in the therapeutic effects. Silver and platinum are both known to have a cooling effect, while gold and copper tend to be warming.

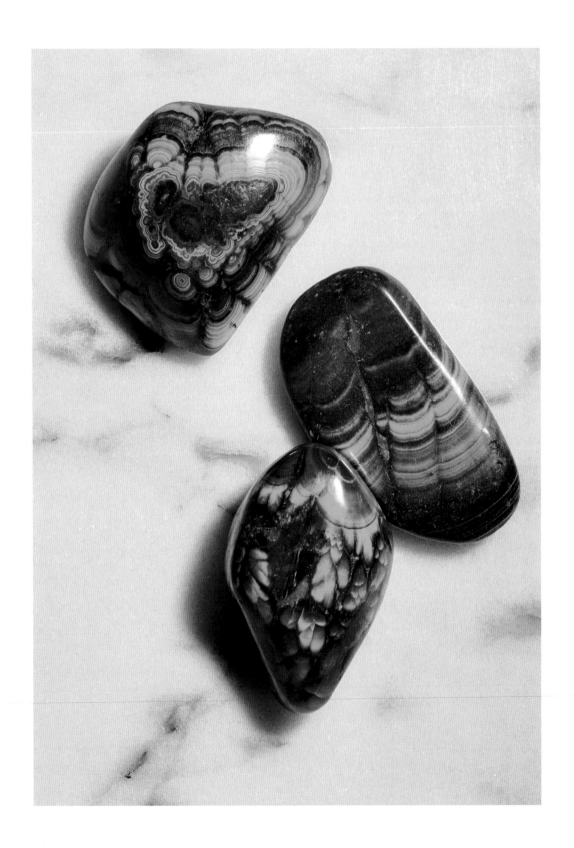

Ideally, you want the stone to have direct contact with your skin. For this reason, rings are said to be more effective when the setting is open at the back, just as shorter necklaces are most effective because they touch skin rather than fabric. That said, a stone's healing properties can be felt through thin wool, cotton, linen, and hemp, but to get the optimal effect, steer clear of synthetic fabrics such as polyester or nylon and from wearing a stone over more than two layers of clothing.

MATTERS OF THE HEART

Whether you're looking to find love, recovering from a broken heart, or just hoping to open your heart to new experiences, there's a crystal or gemstone for that. Here are a few single stones that you may want to combine in one piece of jewelry to accelerate finding a mate—or expedite your ability to love and value yourself:

WATERMELON TOURMALINE

The pink in this stone ushers in healing, while the green represents a fresh start.

KUNZITE

This soothing stone helps you turn your attention to the future so you can stop dwelling on the past.

AVENTURINE

This stone helps heal childhood wounds that are so deeply buried, you may not even remember them.

ROSE QUARTZ

This stone balances emotions, generates self-confidence, and helps you overcome deep-rooted fears.

MALACHITE

This powerful stone brings up issues of the past and helps to release them. Because it digs deep, don't use it alone. Instead, create a pendant or ring that combines malachite with gentle rose quartz.

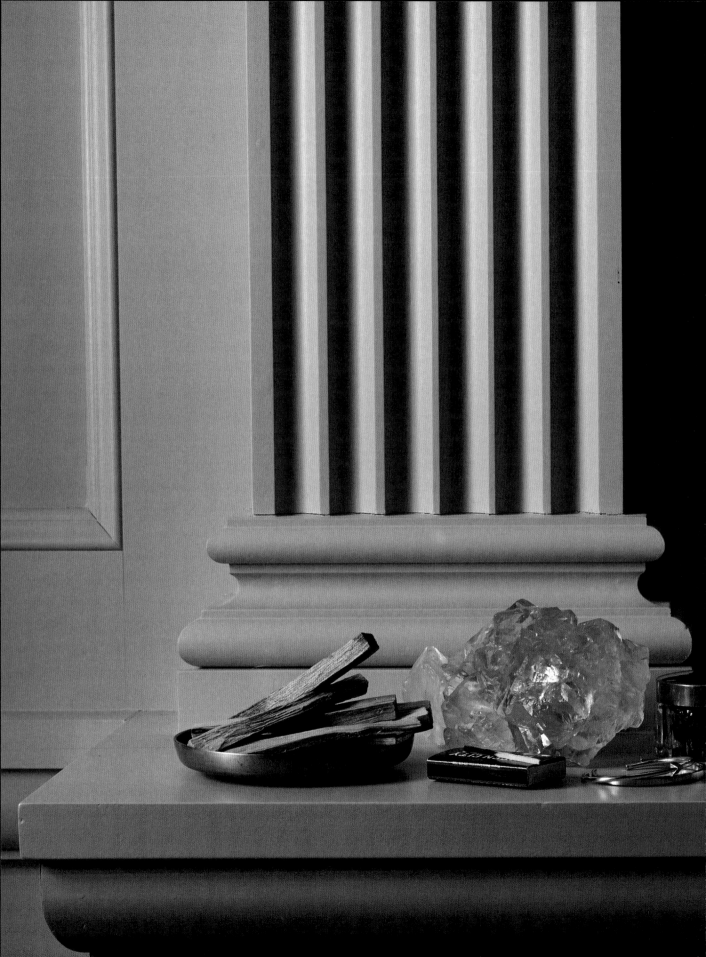

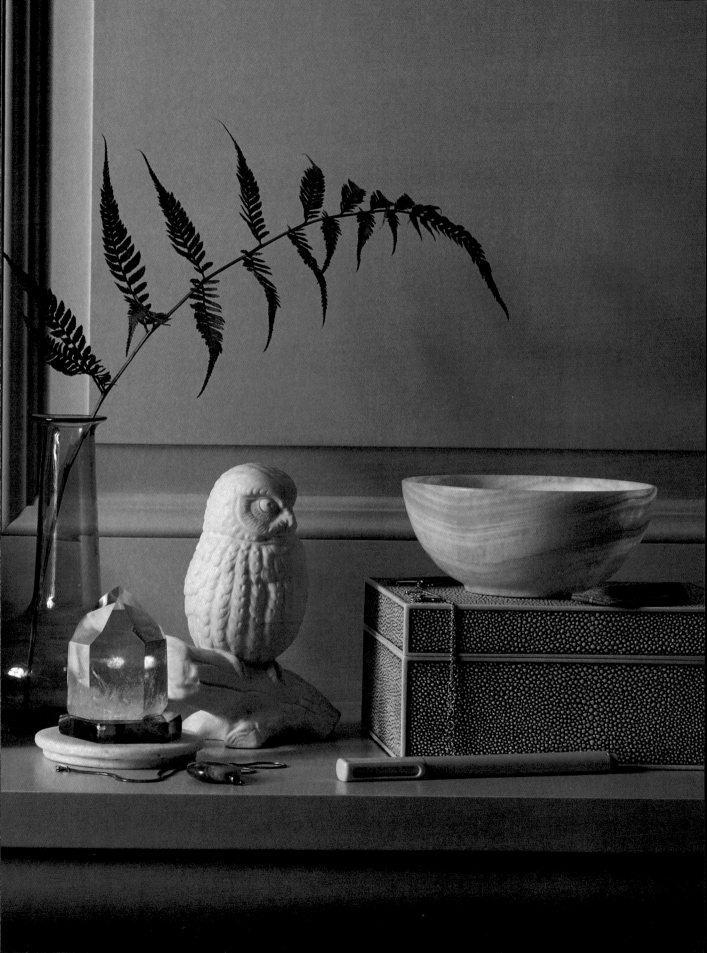

STONES AT HOME

In addition to wearing stones, decorating with them at home will create an inviting atmosphere while also raising the energy level in a particular room. But if you feel your decorating style isn't conducive to stones, or you're concerned that your personal space will end up looking more like an ashram than a tasteful abode, fear not. There are ways to incorporate gemstones and crystals into your home design without compromising your personal aesthetic. A lot of the architects, interior designers, and decorators I've met over the years use crystals and gems as complementary pieces in the home. Whether your abode is classical or more modern, prominently displaying a natural crystal cluster or geode can help anchor a desired energy in a room while also serving as an interesting conversation piece.

CRYSTAL SINGING BOWLS

If you're searching for a decorative crystal bowl that can also be used therapeutically, consider a crystal singing bowl. Made from crushed quartz that is heated to about four thousand degrees in a mold, the bowls are sometimes clear and sometimes frosted and come in a variety of sizes, ranging from 6 to 24 inches in diameter.

What sets the bowls apart from other crystal vessels is that they emit a powerful, pure resonance. The size of the bowl does not necessarily determine its note, although the larger bowls sound lower octaves and notes. The notes—C, D, E, F, G, A, and B—each correspond with one of seven chakras. As with any crystal, some bowls will resonate with you more than others. By listening to the note a bowl emits when you strike the outside with a suede-covered wand and then moving the wand around the bowl in either a clockwise or counterclockwise motion following the sound, you'll get a sense of which tone feels most in line with your individual needs or desires. It takes practice to learn how to hold the stick and move it to get the correct resonance, but it is well worth it: the bowl's music is thought to bring about a positive shift in consciousness.

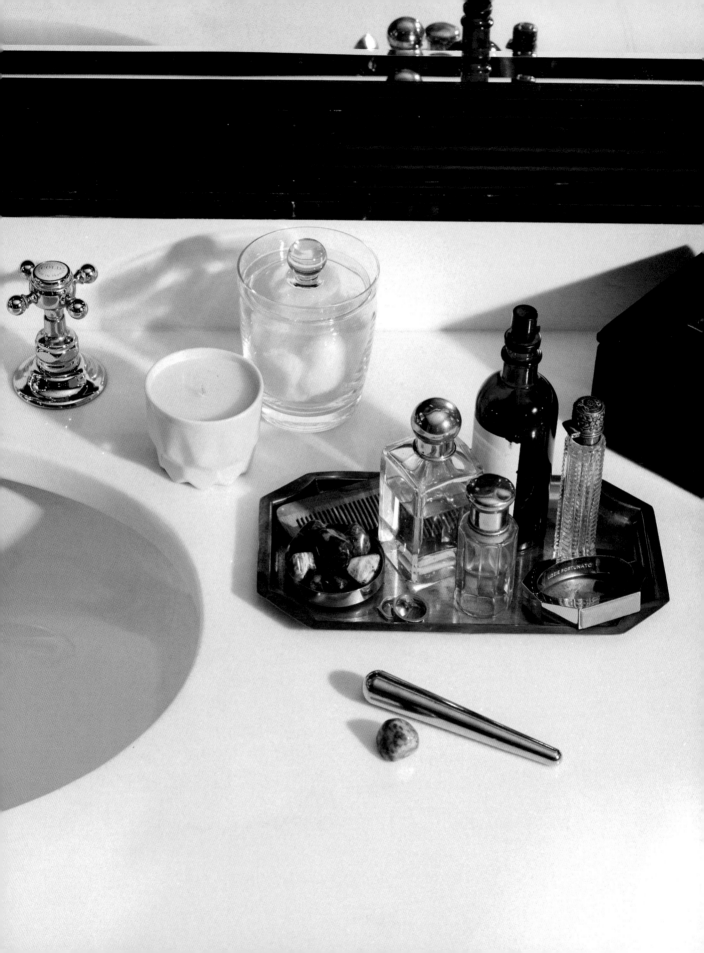

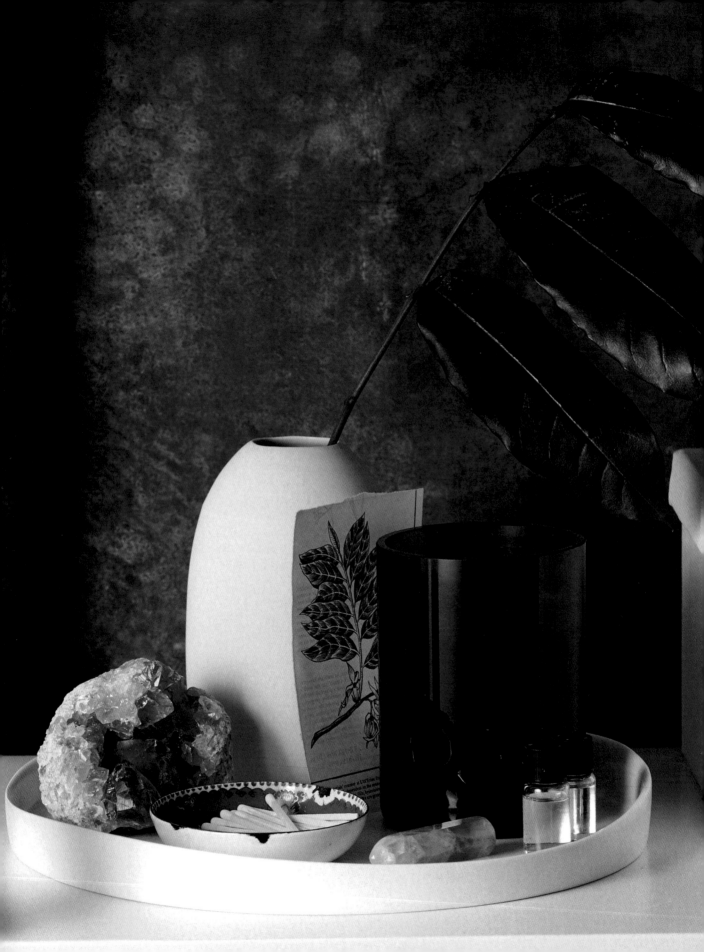

*I've heard of people placing
bowls of tumbled rose quartz on their
bedroom dresser or nightstand to promote
happy, loving relationships.*

If you don't have the space for a large geode, collections of similarly hued stones can easily be placed on a mirrored tray on a coffee table with your favorite books, or in a display case to serve as a focal point in a neutral space or to complement a room's decor. You can also purchase coasters, candleholders, bowls, bookends, boxes, lamps, clocks, and other decorative items made of quartz clusters or geodes.

Stones can also make a splash in the kitchen and bathroom, but don't worry—they won't take up precious counter space. Many modern and well-equipped kitchens feature quartz countertops or other natural materials. Made from one of the hardest minerals on earth, quartz countertops are both durable and pleasing to the eye. But unlike natural-stone slabs, which are mined, these slabs are engineered in a factory. They do contain ground quartz though (about 94 percent), along with polyester resins to bind it and pigments to give it color. A big plus is they're nonporous, so they never need to be sealed—unlike granite, which usually requires a new protective topcoat once a year.

Quartz can also be found in floor tiles that range in both price and color and reflect your personal style. The tiles are available in various shades of pink, white, beige, and gray. Marble, an austere and classic choice, is not only good for the prevention of germs and allergens in the home but is believed to help circulation, skin, and the heart chakra. I've also heard of people adding a little crushed quartz to interior paint when painting rooms in their house. While I haven't tried this, I suggest that if you do, start by adding just a tiny amount, since you want it to have a clearing effect and not an overstimulating one (and stick to living areas rather than bedrooms, because you don't want to jeopardize a good night's sleep).

In addition to choosing quartz to enhance the energy in your home, carefully placing stones throughout the house can provide healing, harmonizing benefits. I keep my rose quartz nearby when I sleep, and I've heard of people placing bowls of tumbled rose quartz on their bedroom dresser or nightstand to promote happy, loving relationships. To generate good dreams for you or a loved one, place a small blue or purple gemstone like holly blue agate or amethyst under your pillow, or a larger one under the bed.

If you have trouble concentrating in your home office, placing fluorite on your desk or around your workspace will aid in bringing structure and divine intellect to the situation or matter at hand. Another great desk stone is glimmering-gold pyrite, which is said to bring crisp, creative financial success and disciplined energy.

Dark stones, such as tourmaline, obsidian, and smoky quartz, have protective qualities, so placing some in large potted plants by or outside your front door may help keep unwanted guests away. I like to keep a few spray bottles of black tourmaline and/or smokey quartz water elixir at the ready throughout my home to spritz as needed to help break up any negative energy while cleansing the aura; if your home has two or more stories, keep one on each floor.

I also suggest keeping plenty of clear quartz—both small crystal quartz apexes and larger clusters—on hand at home, since it has multiple uses. For example, I like to put four crystal quartz apexes in the four corners of a room (with the points facing inward) to improve energy flow. Try keeping the apexes in place for at least an hour and see how you feel afterward. If your heart or mind is racing, put the stones away. If not, keep them there for up to three or four hours. Placing a large clear quartz cluster on a shelf in your home office not only serves as a decorative focal point, but it also helps to promote clarity and order. Another great use for clear quartz is placing one or more small stones or one larger cluster in an area of the home where you meditate or pray regularly to help amplify positive energy.

Speaking of creating a meditation space, I strongly encourage you to do so. Although you can meditate with crystals and gemstones almost anywhere, dedicating a space in your home exclusively for meditation will mark another major step in the ongoing journey of self-discovery through gemstone and crystal healing energy that I hope by now you've chosen to embark upon. It doesn't have to be an entire room, but I have found that having a small space to practice daily helps to slow my racing mind while focusing on a spiritual or divine connection. The space can (and should!) reflect your personal style.

A great starting point is to find an area that is not heavily trafficked and does not house a computer, television, or other electronic gadgets. Make sure to have a space that has some natural light.

As you build your meditation practice, you will most likely be sitting for extended periods of time. Therefore, you might want to consider adding a padded yoga mat or floor pillows, as comfort is key. Additionally, a small, low-to-the-ground table will provide a place for your stones when you're not using them, or you can rest a particular stone there while meditating rather than holding it in your hand. Last, add any artwork, plants, or personal objects that provide you with a sense of peace and serenity while also making the area uniquely yours.

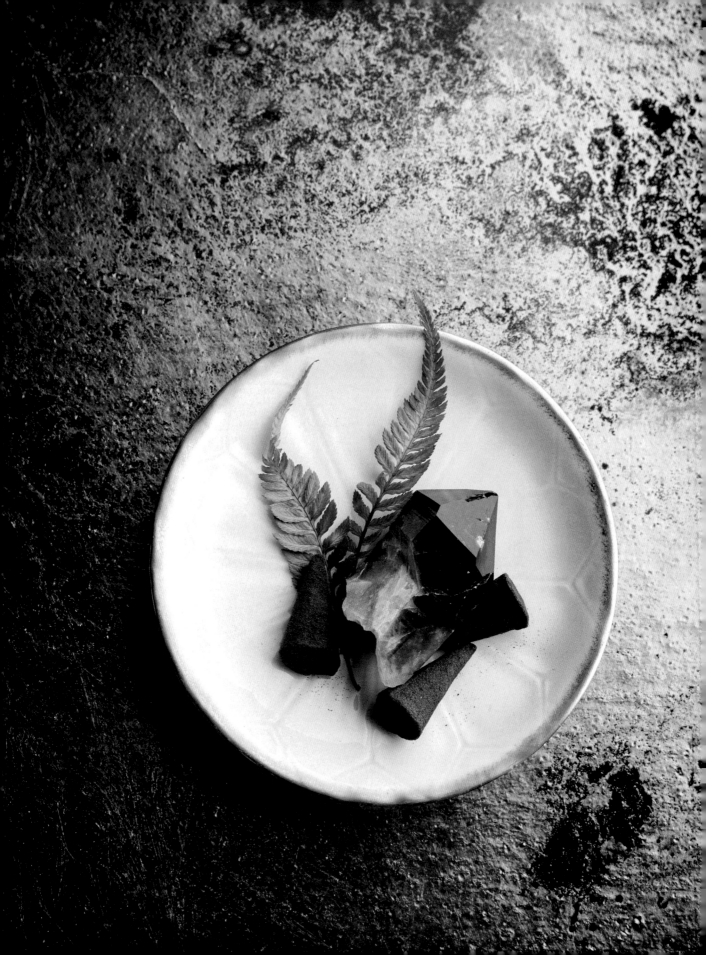

CRYSTAL GRIDS

One way to add a perfect—and purposeful—decorative touch to your meditation space is to create a crystal grid. Crystal grids integrate the power of crystals with sacred geometry to strengthen a focused intention. Archaeologists, anthropologists, and geometricians use the term *sacred geometry* to describe the religious, philosophical, and spiritual beliefs that have sprung up around geometry in various cultures over the course of human history. In a crystal grid, the energy of the stones, the geometric pattern in which you've laid them, and your intention all work as one energy toward a common goal.

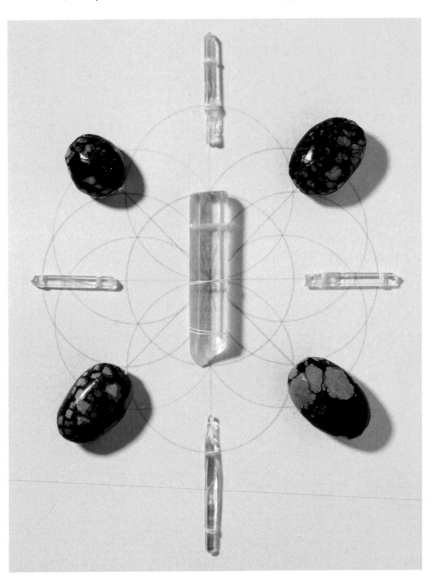

You can find a proliferation of sacred geometry grids online. The grids can be used to help achieve a simple goal, such as enhancing your sleep quality or purification, or for something more elaborate—like personal transformation. The combinations of grids and stones are endless, depending only on your purpose.

You can also purchase crystal grid kits online, making it simple to achieve your intended goal. The art you create by placing the crystals on a specific pattern or grid can be framed to serve as a reminder of your intention, or you can keep it on display for as long as you like before cleaning and reusing the stones on another grid. If you choose to go this route, put your grid on a tray or movable surface, or place it in a spot where you know it will not be disturbed.

Creating a crystal grid is as easy as it is creative. After finding and printing out a grid, simply follow these steps:

1. Decide on your purpose. Do you want to bring more abundance into your life? Enhance your love, peace, and health? Boost creativity? You can create a crystal grid to help manifest your goal.

2. Write your intention on a small piece of paper. When choosing your intention, be as specific as you can, as this will determine which healing stones you choose as part of your grid.

3. Place the piece of paper with your intention at the center of the grid.

4. Gather cleansed and charged crystals and stones that are aligned with your intention. For example, if you are looking to create an abundance grid, use green and gold crystals, such as aventurine, citrine, and pyrite. If you are creating a health and wellness grid, use blue and purple healing stones, such as fluorite, sodalite, and angelite. There are no right or wrong stones; trust your intuition and choose the ones that feel right to you. You'll also need a center or master crystal (see step 6); a crystal point is ideal since it directs your intention straight up into the universe. But any stone will do as long as it's cleansed and charged.

5. Beginning at the outer perimeter of the pattern, place your smaller stones in a geometric pattern.

6. Place the master crystal at the center of the grid on top of the piece of paper on which you've written your intention.

7. To activate the intention, take a quartz crystal apex and, starting from the outside, draw an invisible line between each stone to energetically connect one to the next. Continue until you reach the master crystal.

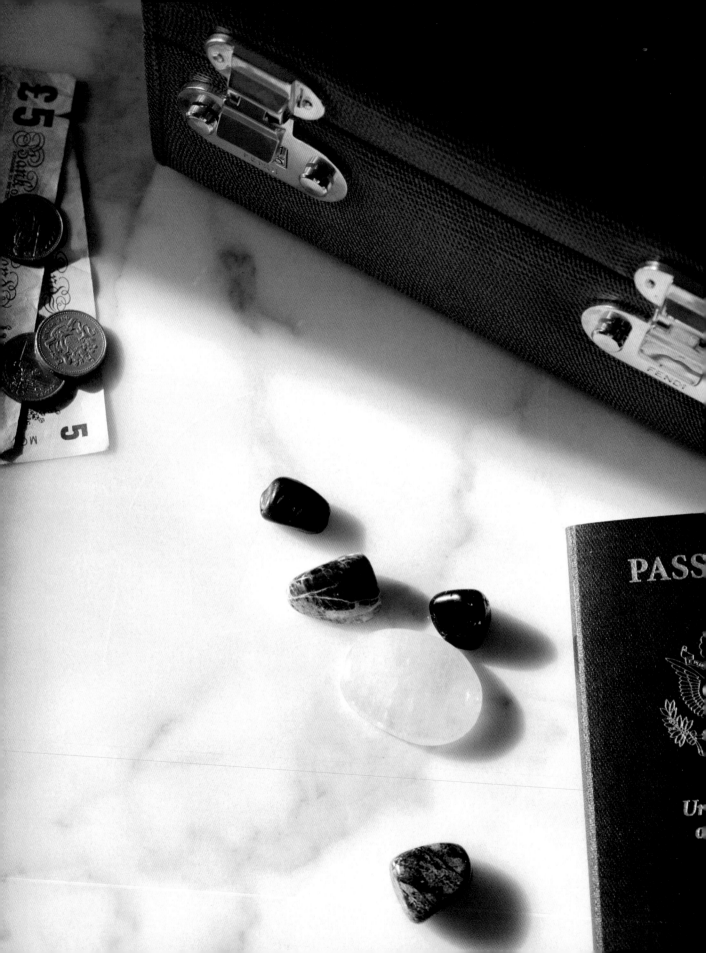

STONES FOR TRAVEL

I'm on the go a lot for my job, and just as I always take a pot of moisturizer, a pair of comfortable flats, and a cashmere wrap with me on the plane, I also make sure to bring a pouch containing my favorite stones.

You wouldn't pack your mobile phone or your laptop in your checked suitcase, would you? Well, the same can be said for your gemstone travel kit. Since certain stones are known to help with everything from travel sickness to anxiety to jet lag, you're going to want to keep them in your carry-on luggage so that you can access them easily while in transit.

What should your kit include? It depends. If you suffer from motion sickness, be sure to take along yellow jasper. I've also found that holding a sodalite stone during the flight helps reduce my fear and anxiety and water retention, as does grasping a malachite stone for protection. For ages, aquamarine has been known as a lucky stone for sailors, but I find that it also makes flying the friendly skies a bit friendlier. If you, like me, get upset at the thought of leaving your loved ones behind when you travel on business, rhodochrosite, a beautiful pink-banded stone known to alleviate emotional upset or stress, is a must. Other fear-reducing crystals, all great for travel, include orange calcite, jade, rose quartz, and onyx. Hold on to whichever stone has the most calming effect on you during takeoff and landing. You can leave it on your lap during the flight, or tuck it in your bra or pocket for safekeeping.

Once you arrive at your destination, holding a clear quartz crystal or black tourmaline while sitting on your hotel-room floor will help clear any energetic imprints left behind from others who have slept there. First, if you can, open all the windows in the room, then hold the clear quartz or tourmaline in your hand and set a concise intention such as "Please remove any traces of previous occupants." Follow this by placing the quartz crystal or tourmaline on a windowsill and leaving the room for an hour or so. When you return, the space should have a warmer, more inviting feel that will make it easier to relax and get to sleep. Gemstones and crystals can also help with jet lag. If you're feeling tired and confused because of a time difference, carry a black tourmaline around with you. If you feel nervous or anxious about being in a new place, celestite will calm the mind and get rid of any worries, while golden topaz is known for releasing tension and stabilizing emotions.

Since I constantly meet new people when I travel, which can be draining, I carry a smoky quartz to protect against any unwanted or negative energy while also energizing myself. Sometimes when I'm feeling homesick, I'll clutch an amethyst, which is a symbol of security as well as serenity—it works to calm my nerves and keep me focused on my purpose while away from home. I've also found beryl to be great for my nerves, or for when I'm missing my husband and son. Charoite, a Russian stone, provides stamina when I'm away for long periods of time, and I've heard it's also good for children who are at boarding school or overnight camp. Another transformative purple stone, sugilite, is believed to be good for nightmares as well as intuition. Historically used as a navigational tool, lodestone, a magnetic and grounding stone, is the perfect stone to round out your travel kit.

Over the years, I've found that crystals and gems are necessary to take along with me on my travels. They help calm me when I'm experiencing more turbulence than normal on a flight, or prevent me from spending the night tossing and turning when sleeping in the guest room of a friend's or relative's home. Stones also help open me up to meeting new people and experiencing things that are outside of my comfort zone.

FEAR OF FLYING

I'm anxious when I fly these days—who isn't? To reduce anxiety,
I rely on a simple hematite-based grounding exercise that you can do
prior to takeoff or midflight to help calm nerves:

1. Take off your shoes so you can feel your feet on the floor.

2. Hold the hematite in the palm of your nondominant hand. Observe the texture of the stone and its weight. Keep the stone in your closed palm and concentrate on its energy.

3. Close your eyes and think of something calming or soothing. Allow the stone to ground your emotions. Be present in your body and aware of how firmly your feet are on the floor.

4. Now visualize any anxiousness leaving your body. Breathe out the energy with each exhale.

5. Open your palm and allow the hematite to absorb any unwanted energy from your mind. Imagine the stone taking in any anxiety and sealing it away.

6. Take two or three deep, cleansing breaths and open your eyes. Tuck the hematite away in a pocket or carry-on.

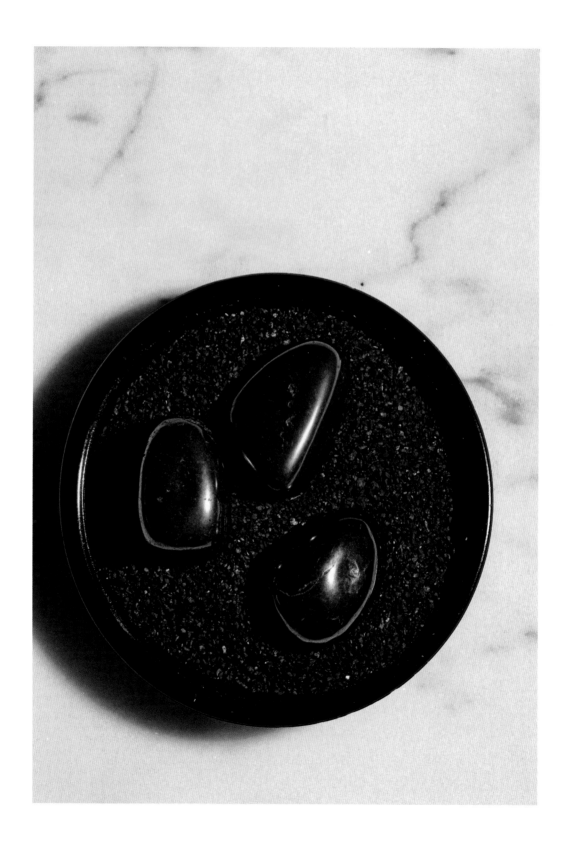

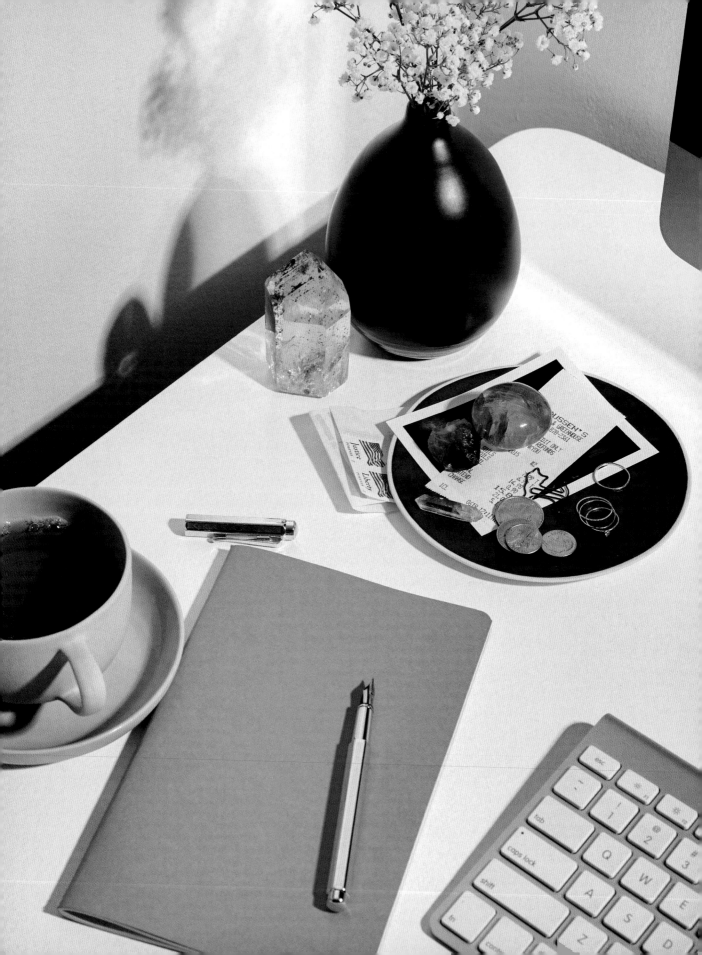

STONES AT WORK

Since your "office"—whatever that may be in the context of your life—is a place where you spend large portions of your time, it's especially wonderful to be able to incorporate crystals and gems into your work life to help keep it happy and vibrant.

I've often found that having a few stones on my desk helps me to de-stress when tensions run high. Simply seeing them there or holding one in my hand when I'm on a high-pressure conference call helps to dissipate stress and keep me on point. I also like to gift my colleagues with crystals when they stay late to help on a project or they receive a much-deserved promotion, and I include a note explaining the crystal's healing properties along with a heartfelt message. Giving stones as gifts is a nice way to spread positive energy throughout your workspace. There are so many ways to surround yourself with the energy of crystals and gems at work, from providing support and creative stimulation to helping you communicate more clearly with coworkers. The following are some crystals and gems that can be of benefit in the workplace, depending on your needs.

ENERGY AND MOTIVATION

Lacking energy and motivation can directly impact your work productivity as well as your bottom line.

Calcite: A great energy amplifier

Carnelian: Increases positive feelings, drive, confidence, and motivation

Green moss agate: Increases hope and optimism and improves self-esteem and self-confidence

LEADERSHIP

Good leadership is essential for any business.

Green aventurine: Reinforces leadership qualities and decisiveness and helps push you outside of your comfort zone

Golden beryl: Invokes the celestial Golden Ray of knowledge and learning to stimulate the higher mind and enable the brain to function more efficiently

Chrysoberyl: Encourages self-discipline, self-control, ambition, and independence and brings to light hidden talents

Amethyst: Helps keep you calm; works with your intuition

CLEAR THINKING

*Keeping a clear head and focusing on what is
important will take you far in the business world, whether you're
a sole proprietor or the CEO of a Fortune 500 company.*

Kyanite: Increases capacity for logical thought, helps clear chakras

Lapis lazuli: Encourages clarity and objectivity; helps give you strength

Chrysocolla: Encourages answers or solutions to become clear

CREATIVITY

*Even a successful business needs constant refreshing, which is
why creativity is an important trait to possess on the job.*

Carnelian and/or citrine: Encourages creative thinking and manifesting
    TIP: Place one under each foot while typing up a big
    presentation or sales pitch.

Rhodochrosite: Stimulates the mind and enhances creativity

Tiger's eye: Releases blocked creativity

ABSORBING/ADAPTING TO NEW IDEAS

*Resisting new ideas has been the downfall of many a successful worker;
these stones are known to help you stay agile and tech-savvy.*

Fluorite: Assists in absorbing new ideas

Blue chalcedony: Opens the mind to novel concepts and helps you to
    accept new situations

Citrine: Encourages you to explore every avenue to find solutions

PUBLIC SPEAKING, COMMUNICATION, AND TEAMWORK

*Clear communication and an all-for-one mentality
can help you stand out from the pack.*

Aquamarine: Removes communication blocks and helps you to deal
    with difficult situations

Amazonite: Dispels negative energy and improves confidence and
    communication
    TIP: Tuck one in your jacket pocket, bra, or shoe before a presentation.

Sodalite: Promotes harmony, trust, and unity of purpose between
    group members

PROTECTION

In a competitive environment filled with recycled air, computers, and draining coworkers, you can use all the protection you can get.

Malachite: Protects against electromagnetic emanations from computers
TIP: Keep one on your desk between you and your screen.
Smoky quartz: Shields you from the energy of negative or emotionally draining people
Agate: Shields you from those who don't wish you well and helps makes them aware of what they are doing

For me, it's become clear that working with crystals and gemstones is a journey that I will continue throughout my lifetime. As we live in a complicated, ever-changing world, I find that using stones in the most basic way (holding them in my hand or placing them on my heart, in my shoes, or in a bath) is a great way to comfort, soothe, ground, protect, and even reconnect. If you take away anything from this book, it's that we are energetic beings who subtly resonate with crystal and gemstone vibrations just as we do with planet Earth. You don't really need to think about it as much as you need to feel it. It's that simple.

A BETTER DAILY COMMUTE

Sitting in traffic or standing in a packed commuter train or bus on the way to or from work can be stressful. In her book *Crystal Energy: 150 Ways to Bring Success, Love, Health, and Harmony into Your Life,* author Mary Lambert suggests keeping an amber stone in your car to maintain a supportive atmosphere. Sometimes called the "honey stone" because it's soft and warm to the touch, amber is known to have a calming energy that absorbs negativity. Place it on the dashboard or in the glove compartment. Envision the stone creating a ring of gold energy around the car that protects you from harm. Cleanse the stone every few months to keep it working for you. If you commute by public transportation, carrying an amber stone can have a similarly protective effect.

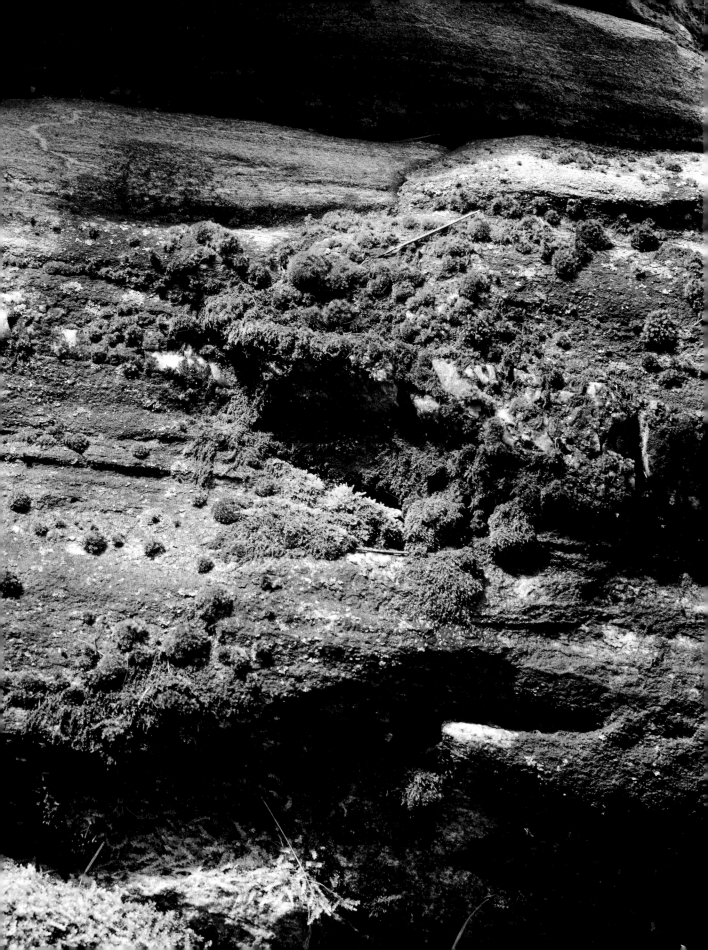

ACKNOWLEDGMENTS

This book was a collaboration of many talented people, all of which helped make *Elemental Energy* possible, starting with my writer, copilot, and fearless trooper, Michele Shapiro, who took on this project helping me to disseminate and decode piles of books and articles on the science and mystery behind these magical crystals and stones. I'm so grateful for your perseverance and wonderful job in helping me to tell my story. And, of course, Camille Trinchillo, who has been my gemstone and crystal advisor since day one—who's generously passed on her knowledge, love, and passion for stones—I could not have done this without you.

My publisher, Claudia Riemer Boutote, who turned an idea and concept into a reality. Her vision, intuition, and belief gave life to this book. Thank you for allowing me this opportunity; I am truly honored.

To Alice Gao, thank you for your dedication to creating thoughtful, stunning photographs, capturing rich moments for everyone to enjoy and immerse themselves in. And our stylist, Kira Corbin, thank you for your integrity and for creating a timeless, modern sensibility.

To Libby Edelson, a great editor with wonderful instincts, thank you for your direction and patience.

To Adrian Morgan, Terri Leonard, and the HarperElixir Team—thank you for your efforts and including me in your process (learning curve and all)!

And Emily Wardwell, thank you for answering my e-mails and bringing visual direction and life into this book, exceeding all expectations.

To Demi Mitchell, for being a fantastic sounding board with great artistic style.

Amanda Birnbaum, for the lovely illustration and always stepping in at a moment's notice.

And Ann Marie Climi, for always bringing consistent and concise expertise to the table.

Estelle Leeds, thank you for answering my questions and always providing amazing help.

And Sara Arnell, for generously giving us the perfect serendipitous setting to shoot in.

My good friend, Michelle Redden, thank you for being my life coach and cheerleader!

A special thanks to Henrik Daniel Gaardsal, Dr. Yury Kronn, Yamil Sarabia, Jill Cohen, and Amber Petrovich.

And to my family, Karen, James, and Van. Thank you for not only being a part of this book but also for all of your unconditional support (you can now take down all the missing wife, mom, and business partner signs). In all seriousness, thank you for your constant patience, love, and support during this process; I could not have done this without you. James, thank you for being my Rock!

Mom, thank you from the bottom of my heart for working, growing, and learning with me throughout the years! Van, hopefully you are too young to remember any of this!

And last but not least, I would like to thank God—I do not recall this being on my bucket list—thank you for opening my eyes.

RESOURCE GUIDE

CRYSTALS AND GEMSTONES
Exquisite Crystals
http://www.exquisitecrystals.com
360-573-6787

Emily Gems
http://crystal-cure.com
937-508-4482

AstroGems
http://www.astrogems.com
1-888-833-4225

Rockstar NYC
http://rockstarcrystalsmanhattan.com
212-675-3065

Madagascar Stones
http://www.madagascargemstones.com/about_us
415-418-0641

Bliss Crystals
https://www.etsy.com/shop/BlissCrystals

Kashmir Blue
http://kashmirblue.com

COLLOIDALS
Purist Colloids
https://www.purestcolloids.com

PEARL POWDER
Jing Herbs Pearl Powder
www.jingherbs.com

ELIXIRS
Pegasus Products
http://www.pegasusproducts.com
303-652-3424

Ascended Earth
http://www.ascendedearth.com
1-888-800-2057
1-610-482-4817

SPECIALTY SALTS
The Spice Lab
http://shop.thespicelab.com

HERBS AND CARRIER OILS
Monterey Bay Spice Company
http://www.herbco.com

BIRCH CHIPS
Scentsible Crafts
http://scentsible-crafts.myshopify.com

TESLA PLATES
Purple Plates
http://www.purpleplates.com
860-830-9069

For all other ingredients, I recommend purchasing from your local health food market or Whole Foods and buying organic whenever possible.

INDEX

Page numbers in *italic* indicate illustrations.

CREDITS

Additional Photography and Illustrations

p. ix, Kristin walking on the beach: Christian Tay

p. xi, Kristin and Karen: Matt Albiani

pp. 22 and 137, chakra illustrations: Amanda Birnbaum

p. 110, Therme Vals: Courtesy 7132 Hotel Vals

p. 191, Irene Neuwirth One-of-a-Kind Necklace Set with Mixed Stones: Courtesy Irene
   Neuwirth

p. 202, crystal grid: Carrie Borgen

p. 227, about the author: Christian Tay

ABOUT THE AUTHOR

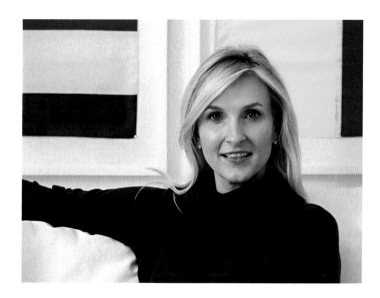

Kristin Petrovich is the cofounder and creator of själ skincare, a gemstone-
and precious-mineral-infused bioactive cosmetic line that integrates ancient
Eastern medicines with innovative Western biotechnology. For over a decade,
Kristin has studied and embraced insights from the worlds of Chinese, Tibetan,
ayurvedic, homeopathic, and vibrational energy medicine. Kristin resides in
Greenwich, Connecticut, with her husband, James, and son, Van.

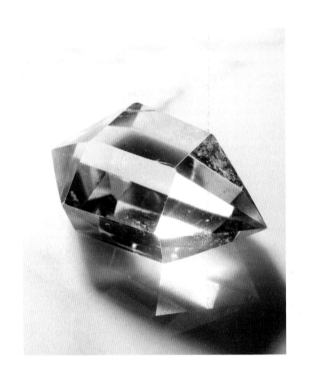